SUFFERING...With A Smile!

Copyright ©2016 Clevon Harris

International Standard Book Number:

ISBN 10   1523752130

ISBN 13   9781523752133

LCCN:

Printed in the United States of America
To order additional copies please contact
Miracleintentions@yahoo.com
4 decades? Youtube: Miracleintentions@MyGodReigns
www.fightingsickness.com
Amazon.com/author/clevonharris

1. Water: Drink 8-12 cups daily.
2. Dark Green Vegetables: Eat 3-4 times a week.
3. Whole Grains: Eat 2 or 3 times daily.
4. Beans and Lentils: Eat a bean meal once a week.
5. Fish: Eat 3-4 oz of quality fish a week (page 80).
6. Fruit (Berries are #1): Eat 2-3 servings daily.
7. Soy, nuts, seeds and yogurt are top health foods.

DISCLAIMER:

The information in this publication has been written and recorded as possible natural solutions in helping others achieve better health. However, this information can also be very helpful to anyone who desires to eat healthier, feel better and have more energy. This information is in no way said to be a cure for any ailment. Everyone is different, so individual results may vary. When you are trying to achieve certain results from a diet, you must be dedicated and willing to sacrifice certain foods that you may ordinarily desire. Some foods may have to be either cut back or totally cut out of your diet. It is also very important to watch what you drink. Certain liquids will destroy vitamins and minerals the body needs. *A healthy fasting regime can help boost immune system, brain health etc.* Pg 11, 47

Have you ever thought about preparing some of your foods without a constant use of a microwave? On page 204, I explain why I asked that question. The information found in this publication is based upon my studies, experiments and opinions. I am not a doctor. Be sure to always consult with your doctor or healthcare physician before changing any diet. **When** we eat **some** foods **is** vital. Pg 73, 151

Note: I take organic turmeric powder because it is easier for me to use than the raw root. Turmeric is not easily absorbed. For better absorption, combine equal amounts of turmeric, olive oil and a dash of ground pepper. I take **1-2** tbsp daily/as needed for pain or back pain. See pg 191. Protein, probiotics, exercise and rest increase **dopamine**. Pg 157, 212

Table of Contents

SUFFERING WITH A
SMILE

There is NO medicine like hope!! Miracles do happen!

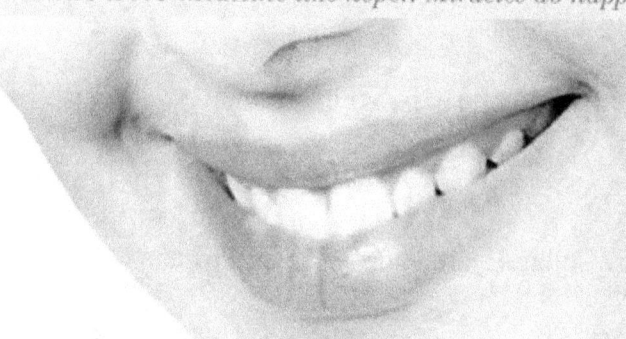

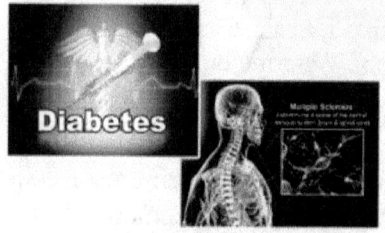

"We never know what struggle or battle a person may be going through! Just because the person we see is smiling, laughing or appears to be doing fine... does not mean they really are."

CLEVON HARRIS

Mr. Harris was featured in a special Athens News Courier edition featuring "100 people who make a difference."

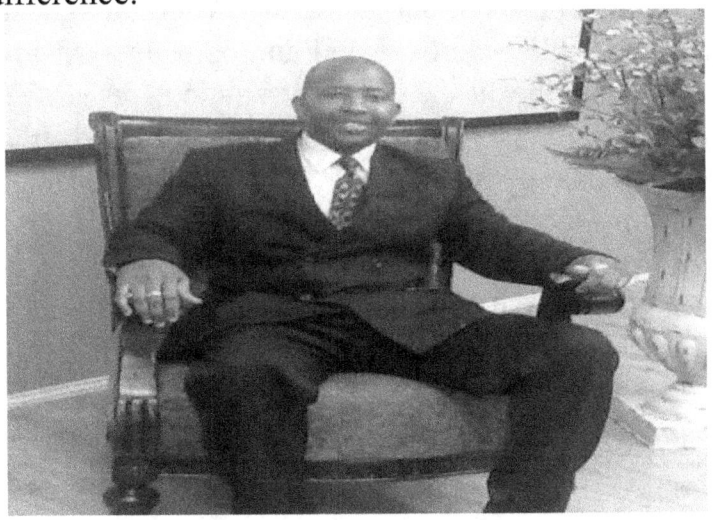

After having been diagnosed with MS I have been inspired, encouraged and helped by his published books. There are indeed many great things ahead for this young man as he continues to allow the hand of almighty God to direct his every move and orchestrate his every endeavor! I am personally waiting with great anticipation for his next body of work!

~ Karen Prater. Newport News, VA

Author of *"Dancing While in The Valley"* and *"Are You Suited & Ready For Battle? Every Believer's Guide to Spiritual Warfare"*

I know Clevon has studied health for a long time and he has helped himself as well as many others improve their health. I often find myself asking him health questions because I value his opinion.

~James McElroy. Pulaski, TN

Mr. Harris has a compelling desire to see others reap the benefits of being healthy. After a diagnosis with Multiple Sclerosis, and an enduring stint in a wheelchair, he has vigorously studied, researched and meticulously tested products and foods that assist the body in healing. Prescribed medicines, oftentimes only make you feel better for a short duration. He will provide concise information to maintain your health. Wouldn't it be wonderful to eliminate some or most of your medicine closet?

~Tamara H. Boman. Birmingham, AL
Host of "Real Talk with THB", Author of *"And Still Daddy's Girl"*, *"Karma Sings The Married Man's Blues"* and *"Flesh And Spirit"*.

I enjoyed *My MS Success* by Mr. Harris and I anticipate the release of his next book! By keeping God and prayer in your life you can achieve anything!

~Thersa Smith. Athens, AL

I call Mr. Harris the "Ambassador" because he goes around trying to help so many people. I really appreciate his advice. I read his first two books and look forward to reading his third.

~Lisa Gardner Peoples. Evanston, Illinois

Mr. Harris is more than just an author of great publications, he is also a friend. His motivational words and encouragement have lifted my spirits throughout my painful ordeal. He has reminded me that no matter how seemingly unbearable the pains of my illness, I am stronger, can endure much and overcome anything.

~Kimberly Brown. Athens, AL

I've known Mr. Harris for years. I was in need of help with my everyday stressed out life and I decided to contact him. It all started with a change in my living and eating lifestyle. I now feel like I've been revitalized.

~Sharon Pressnell. Athens, AL

Your body is a collection of cells which depend on oxygen in order to sustain life. Being able to think and move require your body to possess oxygen. A decrease of oxygen in the blood can possibly lead to respiratory problems and if prolonged can cause cell dysfunction and death of brain cells. Eat foods high in fatty acids, exercise frequently for better blood circulation, consume antioxidants (this will help your body utilize oxygen more efficiently by dilating blood vessels) and breathe fresh air daily.
Top antioxidants: *berries, beans, green vegetables, cranberries, prunes, apples, cocoa, nuts, red wine*

DEDICATION

Suffering With A Smile was on my agenda years before I published *Your Health And Healing*. At first I started to just let this title go and never start a third publication. After my second bout with MS, the desire to complete *Suffering With A Smile* was once again burning in my heart. I was led to move forward and finish this publication. All of us have something in our lives that we struggle with. Our struggles will vary from person to person and all of our struggles are not visible. People need someone that understands them and someone they can talk to during their trying and very difficult times.

I dedicate this book to anyone that is battling or struggling with their health/ailment. As you read this book, rest assured knowing that you are not alone. If you have an illness, been diagnosed with a disease or even sometimes feel like an outcast, I understand what you may be going through. We are in this battle together. We are more similar to one another than we are different. Stay strong and always believe because miracles really do happen. Hold your head up and prepare to move forward. It's not how you start, it's how you finish. Giving up is not an option. This publication is dedicated to anyone that may be *Suffering With A Smile!*

Clevon Harris

Eccl 7:17 *"neither be thou foolish: why shouldest thou die before thy time?"*

INTRODUCTION

Hello! My name is Clevon Harris, author of *My MS Success* and *Your Health And Healing*. In this publication, I plan is to be as direct and to the point as quick as possible. I understand that when people are seeking help, they want answers that they can easily comprehend. If certain foods will help with certain conditions, I will tell you what the certain foods are. I feel that the quicker you receive the information you are seeking, the quicker you will be on your way to achieving optimal health. Many words in this publication are typed in italics/bold because I want you to notice them. I'll often direct you to other pages if the information is related.

On the cover of this publication you may have noticed that cancer, diabetes and multiple sclerosis appear to be my three main objectives. Cancer has damaged, devastated and taken many of my close friends. Diabetes attempt to overwhelm my family. Multiple sclerosis has attacked me. Millions suffer from these vile diseases every single day. I thank God that I have great success stories that involve these three disease/ailments. I will be sharing them with you. While reading this publication you will find information that can help assist sufferers of many other health ailments as well. It bothers me when I look at TV commercials, watch the news or hear and read about the difficult struggles people have to endure. I try my best to share knowledge I have acquired during my years of study, trial and error. In *Your Health And Healing,* I shared a pH balance food chart with alkaline/enzyme rich foods on page 37. It's time to reclaim your health and the genuine smile you once had. It's time to smile with confidence in the presence of adversity. I pray this publication will be a blessing to you or someone you love. This book covers many foods, fruits and vegetables that aid our health. Studies have shown that actual fruits and vegetables are healthier than their supplement versions. Our body can heal best while we are sleep. Always keep in mind that "Life is more enjoyable when you are healthy!"

HUMAN EMOTIONS

Before we get started I would like to take a look at something that we all have...EMOTIONS! You may not know, you may have never been taught but our emotions have a significant impact on our health. When we get mad or angry, that emotion can effect and weaken our liver. If we get scared or fearful, that emotion can weaken our kidney. If or when stricken with grief, that emotion can weaken our lungs. When dealing with stress, be advised that it can weaken our heart and our brain. If you find yourself worried all the time keep in mind that worry can weaken our stomach. It makes perfect sense to me that after many people are diagnosed with a serious disease their health appears to spiral downhill faster. Emotions have consumed them and unfortunately everyone's mindset is not strong. It has been reported that the average human uses around 10% of their brain. What are we doing with the remaining 90%? The mind is a terrible thing to waste and a strong mind is a very powerful asset to good health. Think positive. There is NO medicine like hope! Miracles do happen!

Psalms 27:1
The Lord is my light and my salvation; whom shall I fear? the Lord is the strength of my life; of whom shall I be afraid?

Psalms 27:3
Though an host should encamp against me, my heart shall not fear: though war should rise against me, in this will I be confident.

Ecclesiastes 7:9
Be not hasty in thy spirit to be angry: for anger resteth in the bosom of fools.

Matthew 6:34
Take therefore no thought for the morrow: for the morrow shall take thought for the things of itself...

Colossians 3:8
But now ye also put off all these; anger, wrath, malice, blasphemy, filthy communication out of your mouth.

In the disclaimer, I mention that a **healthy fasting regime** can boost the immune system, brain health and more. Many religions practice fasting. It helps create an environment in which healing can occur. Fasting initiates the body's healing mechanisms, so **any ailment** may show improvement. It takes a lot of work to digest our meals. It's estimated that 65% of our body's energy has to be directed to digestive organs after a big meal. Also see page 47 and 61.

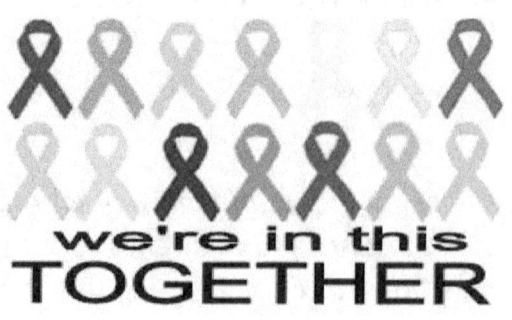

we're in this
TOGETHER

CANCER

Let's start things off by talking about cancer for a minute. Cancer has attacked so many men, women and children. The cancer diagnosis rate continues to rise. Cancer has attacked many of my close and dear friends. I've seen cancer attack and this is why I developed an even stronger desire to help fight this disease. Please take a moment and allow me to share a few of my personal cancer stories with you.

I was talking with a loving Christian lady at her grandchild's birthday party. She was a blessing to be around. She was always smiling and full of joy. While conversing with her we happen to divert our attention to the importance of good health. She informed me that she had been diagnosed with cancer for quite some time. It was 2002 and I had just began studying health awareness. I was ready to help her any way that I could. Less than a month later, I was in attendance at her funeral. She passed away....due to cancer. It was a sad day, I felt very helpless but I felt comfort knowing that she knew Jesus. My goal on trying to help others fight their ailment intensified. Her death helped inspire me.

CANCER

2005, just 3 years later I found myself attending another funeral. At this funeral I was holding and consoling a friend of mine as she and I both were grieving the loss of one of our close, young and Christian friends. He had just passed away....due to cancer. In such a short time, it was another death.

Lets fast forward to the year 2009. I found myself attending the funeral of my friend I was consoling at the funeral I previously mentioned. She had passed away...due to cancer. If that wasn't enough, in 2012 I lost a great friend that ran track with me in high school, built my website, taught me most of what I know about computers and was always willing to lend a helping hand....due to cancer. In 2014 one of my older cousins passed away due to guess what...you guessed it....cancer! These are some of the incidents where I have lost loved ones due to cancer. I can't remember seeing or hearing any of them complain. They all wore big beautiful smiles but they were all suffering. It appears that every time I turn around, cancer has found another victim. It is definitely time to fight back.

If you know someone that has been diagnosed or battling cancer, please share the *cancer fighting* and *high risk cancer foods* I have listed ahead with them. The list ahead is even more diverse than the list I shared with a lady in 2003 I consulted with that had just been diagnosed with cancer. She took the list very serious, remained dedicated to it and her doctor eventually informed her that the cancer was gone. To this day, she has been cancer free. I will first start off with the foods to add to your diet to help fight cancer. As you continue to read you will find that certain foods help fight **specific** type cancers. *Cancer can't live in an alkaline rich body.*

Fruit, Vegetables (fruit:best 30-45 min after meal)

1. *Almonds*

2. *Apples* (Especially red apples.)

3. *Avocados* (Provide more potassium than bananas and they are useful in treating breast, prostate and certain causes of liver cancer.)

4. *Beets* (Fight inflammation & lower blood pressure.)

5. *Blueberries* (Berries in general fight cancer.)

6. *Broccoli*

7. *Brussels Sprouts*

8. *Cabbage*

9. *Cantaloupe*

10. *Cauliflower*

11. *Carrots* (May help fight or reduce a wide range of cancers including lung, mouth, throat, stomach, intestine, bladder, prostate and breast.)

12. *Celery*

13. *Chili Pepper* (Can help prevent certain cancers such as stomach cancer)

14. *Cranberries*

15. *Garlic* (Eating garlic regularly (especially raw) can help fight the risk of stomach cancer and colon rectal cancer.)

16. *Ginger*

17. *Grapes*

18. *Grapefruits* (Can help fight breast cancer.)

19. *Graviola Tea*

20. *Honeydew Melon*

21. *Jalapenos* (Same as chili peppers.)

22. *Kale*

23. *Lemons*

24. *Mushrooms* (Maitake, Reishi, Agaricus blazei Murill, Shiitake and Coriolus Versicolor. Each type can help fight cancer and build a *stronger immune system.*)

25. *Onions*

26. *Oranges*

27. *Papaya* (best eaten 4-5 hours after a meal)

28. *Prunes* (drink 1 to ½ cup prune juice in morning)

29. *Radish*

30. *Raspberries*

31. *Seaweed*

32. *Spinach*

33. *Squash*

34. *Strawberries*

35. *Sweet potatoes*

36. *Tomatoes* (Lycopene found in tomatoes can kill mouth cancer cells and reduce the risk of breast, prostate, pancreas and colon rectal cancer. Due to their healthy fats, consume some avocados or olive oil with your tomatoes for better absorption.)

37. *Whiskey* (I drink very little whiskey. Page 26)

38. *Yams*

Herbs & Spices

1. Rosemary

2. Turmeric can help fight bowel and colon cancer.

3. Parsley

Liquids

1. Red wine (Drink in moderation.)

2. Soy Products could help prevent both breast and prostate cancer.

3. Green Tea may help reduce the risk of stomach, lung, colon, rectum, liver and pancreas cancer.

4. Black Tea can reduce the risk of cancer, stroke, lower cholesterol, blood pressure & aid gut flora.

Grains, Etc

1. Fiber

2. Figs & Dates (Nutrient similar **Bible health fruit.**)

3. Flax Seeds can protect against colon cancer and heart disease.

4. Nuts can suppress the growth of cancers, Brazil nuts help fight prostate cancer.

5. Whole Grains

Fish

Fish high in Omega 3 fatty acids such as mackerel, tuna, salmon and sardines help fight cancer.

CANCER

POSSIBLE HIGH RISK CANCER CAUSERS

1. Genetically-modified organisms (GMOs)

2. Processed meats: bacon, sausage, bologna, lunch meats, hot dogs, ham, liver, high fat meats

3. Unless your fruits and vegetables are organic or verified to be pesticide-free, they could potentially be a major cancer risk.

4. Carbonated drinks can acidify the body and feed cancer cells. *Sugar feeds every cell in the body.*

5. *Artificial sweeteners such as aspartame* can help cause many types of problems such as birth defects and cancer. Sucralose, saccharin and other artificial sweeteners have been reported as high risk cancer causers. *Aspartame can cause seizures, ADHD etc.*

6. Microwave popcorn. I have read that the bags the popcorn is sealed in, are lined with chemicals that have been linked to causing infertility, liver, testicular, and pancreatic cancers. Not to mention infertility. (*Cancer cells need glucose for energy.*)

7. Hydrogenated oils: These oils are found in many of our foods. They can be the cause of many health problems including cancer. Find the chapter titled NOTES and go to page 148 for more information.

8. Smoked fish and highly salted foods may raise stomach, colon, ovarian and prostate cancer risk. Alcohol, tobacco, mayonnaise, margarine, butter and coffee should all be consumed in moderation.

If fighting cancer, keep in mind the consumption and your preparation/cooking methods of the foods that are listed ahead.

Eggs
- Yolks and whites should be cooked solid.
- Any foods that may have raw eggs in them

Dairy Products
- Milk, yogurt, cheese and any other dairy products that are not pasteurized
- Bleu cheese, cheeses with blue veins or soft cheeses
- Queso, blanco, fresco and other Mexican cheeses

Fruits and vegetables
- Raw alfalfa or other raw vegetable sprouts
- Fresh salsa or salad dressings that are kept in the refrigerated cases of the grocery store
- Fruit and vegetable juices that are not pasteurized

Meat

*Fully cook red meats but do not overcook.

•Eat small portion sizes. 17oz a week is fine.

•Thoroughly cook all meat and seafood.

Other

•Sweets that have creamy fillings
•Raw honey (heat-treated honey only)
•If you eat tofu, cook it for at least 5 minutes

BBQ Grilling Meat And Cancer

BBQ can look so good and delicious with those beautiful grill marks but the downside is *excessive amounts of grilled meat or chicken can increase your risk of developing cancer.* Not only the grilled foods but pan-fried meats at high temperatures as well. Use rosemary to soak up some free radicals.

When very high temperatures break down the amino acid creatine in the meats, a carcinogenic chemical known as heterocyclic amines (HAs) is formed. Anything burnt contains carbon which can lead to cancer. If you have consumed something that had char marks or was burnt in places, eat a tomato or some strong cancer fighter after wards to possibly neutralize the carcinogenic food you just ingested. Burnt food increases free radicals which can lead to cancer. I mentioned a tomato because they are great at destroying free radicals. If you eat food that is grilled or charred, do so in moderation. **(Medium rare steak is considered perfectly cooked.)**

Processed food: A large number of ingredients, with names that you don't recognize, indicates a highly processed food. Virtually every food that comes in a box, bag, jar, or can is processed. Processed food applies to any food that has been altered from its natural state somehow. Processed foods are not necessarily unhealthy all of the time.

Pink...
Breast Cancer

Teal...
Ovarian Cancer

Clear...
Lung Cancer

Purple...
Pancreatic &
Leiomyosarcoma

Orange...
Leukemia

Emerald Green...
Liver Cancer

Periwinkle Blue...
Esophageal &
Stomach Cancer

Black...
Melanoma

Dark Blue...
Colon Cancer

Burgundy...
Multiple Myeloma

Grey...
Brain Cancer

Blue...
Prostate Cancer

Teal/White...
Cervical Cancer

Yellow...
Sarcoma/Bone/
Bladder Cancer

Gold...
Childhood Cancers

Burgundy/Ivory...
Head & Neck Cancer

Lime...
Lymphoma

Peach...
Uterine Cancer

Kelly Green...
Kidney Cancer

Teal/Pink/Blue...
Thyroid Cancer

Lavender...
All Cancers

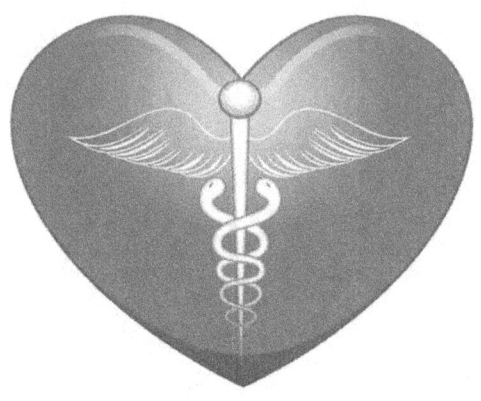

DIABETES

Now, let's talk diabetes. Diabetes can easily be found on my dad's side of the family. My dad, his sister and one of my older sister have all been diagnosed with diabetes. Diabetes is a noteworthy health ailment that can be controlled and it needs to be taken seriously. I discussed diabetes in *Your Health And Healing* so I will try my best to be brief about it in this publication. I believe you will find the information that I discuss in this chapter informative and very beneficial.

Many of the signs of Type 1 and Type 2 diabetes are similar. In both, there is to much glucose in the blood and not enough in the cells of your body. High glucose levels in Type 1 are due to a lack of insulin because the insulin producing cells have been destroyed. Type 2 diabetes occurs when the body's cells become resistant to the insulin that is being produced. As with any disease or ailments, there are usually warning signs. Several of the top warning signs of diabetes are mentioned next.

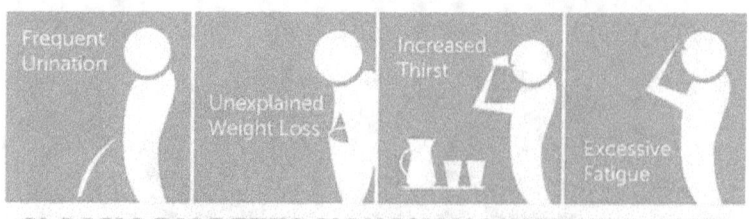

CLASSIC DIABETES SIGNS YOU MUST NOT MISS!

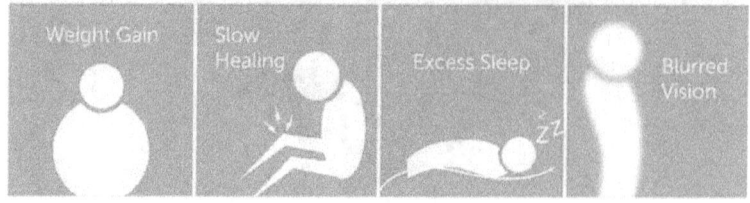

Unquenchable Thirst

Fatigue and Weakness

Losing Weight Without Trying

Frequent Trips to the Bathroom

Tingling or Numbness in Your Hands, Legs or Feet: This symptom is called neuropathy. It occurs gradually over time as *consistently high glucose* in the blood damages the nervous system (often felt in your extremities). Type 2 diabetes is a gradual onset, and people are often not aware that they have it. Neuropathy can very often improve when tighter blood glucose control is achieved. Blurred vision, skin that is dry or itchy, frequent infections or cuts and bruises that take a long time to heal are also signs and symptoms that can occur. If you notice any of these warning signs, please schedule an appointment with your doctor.

Note: 5/plus servings of **white rice** a week can **raise** risk of type 2 diabetes 17%. 2 servings of **brown rice** a week can **decrease** the risk of type 2 diabetes by 11%.

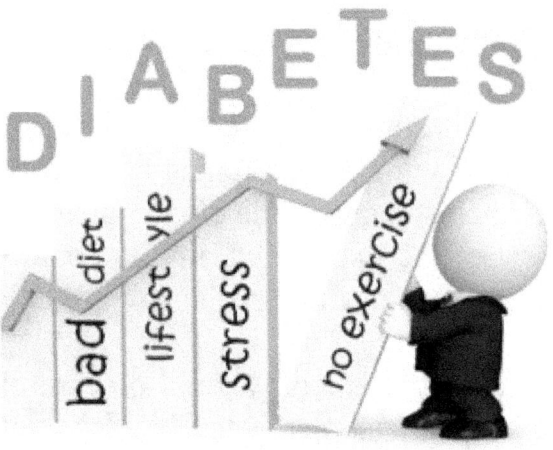

What are some changes a diabetic can do to help improve their health? Exercise, stay hydrated with water, keep a healthy weight, increase fiber intake, watch the carbohydrates, control stress, get quality sleep and eat low glycemic foods (seafood, eggs, yams, beans, corn, non-starchy fruit/vegetables).

Many may know that chromium is a mineral that is very beneficial and necessary for better diabetes management. Some people may be somewhat new to the mineral vanadium. Vanadium can also help assist diabetic patients. I will give a short summary of both chromium and vanadium. I will list some cons and pros of each one as well as natural food sources they are found in. Following that, you will find *Foods That Assist Diabetics.* Diabetic patients should definitely read this. Drink okra water too. It fights diabetes, cholesterol, high blood pressure, is anti-cancer, aids the heart and strengthens *immune system.* Drink on an empty stomach. (Page 27, 92)

Health Importance Of Chromium

Chromium is an essential mineral required for the normal functioning of the human body. Chromium indirectly helps maintain the blood glucose level. A deficiency of the mineral chromium could lead to the symptoms of insulin resistance.

Type 2 diabetic patients should be careful when taking chromium supplements. Excessive intake of chromium supplements can possibly cause glucose intolerance and/or hypoglycemia. It can also cause damage to your genetic materials. *For best results, try to consume healthy foods that naturally contain chromium instead of taking the different chromium supplements.* Next you will find natural foods that contain high amounts of chromium. Many of them are listed ahead:

Brewers Yeast
Brewers yeast is easily one of the best sources of chromium. Two tablespoons of brewers yeast can provide the daily requirements & adequate amount of chromium.

Sweet Potato

Corn

Whole Grains

Meat
Beef, Liver, Poultry, Turkey

DIABETES

Seafood

Oysters, Shellfish

Fruit, Vegetables (fruit:best 30-45 min after meal)

Apple, Banana, Basil Leaves (dry), Beet, Broccoli, Chili (fresh), Garlic, Grape Juice, Green Pepper, Lettuce, Mushroom, Onion, Orange Juice, Spinach and Tomato

Other Diabetic Assistance To Consider

Apple Cider Vinegar, Berberine, Cinnamon

Fenugreek Seeds, Magnesium

Glucose is our most important sugar. It's the body's preferred source of energy. The most concentrated source is honey, followed by dried fruit. (Page 35)

Health Importance Of Vanadium

Vanadium is an essential trace mineral that can be found in shellfish such as shrimp, lobster and crab. Vanadium might play a role in building your bones and teeth. The presence of this mineral in our brain can inhibit cholesterol from forming in our blood vessels because it can inhibit cholesterol synthesis. Vanadium is effective in a lot of chemical reactions that take place in our bodies. Vanadium is found in very small amounts in a wide variety of foods like *dill seed, black pepper, spinach, mushroom, whole grains, cereals, seafood, meats, tomatoes, parsley, vegetable oils, garlic, green beans, corn, carrots, onions and cabbage. Beer, wine and drinks made with artificial sweeteners* also contain vanadium.

Why is vanadium listed in this section? Vanadium may also help maintain healthy glucose and lipid metabolism. Very similar to chromium, people that are diagnosed with diabetes or hyperglycemia are cautioned not to ingest supplemental vanadium to manage their diabetes or hyperglycemia. I've tried to find and study vanadium supplements for many years now. It was reported years ago that vanadium supplements resulted in being toxic to the human body. For that reason you could not purchase them off the shelves. That was years ago and things have now changed. It took a long time for the pill form of vanadium to finally pass. *For the best results, I would suggest natural consumption of vanadium from natural food sources.* Natural is always better and easier absorbed by our body than synthetic.

Cautions and side effects of Vanadium

Vanadium can cause stomach cramping, diarrhea and in some cases green tongue when taken in high dosages. It is possible there could be an interaction between vanadium and chromium so be advised.

If you plan to take extra chromium, it may be best to take it at a different time from taking vanadium supplements. (Tobacco reduces vanadium intake.)

Whiskey (whiskey aka whisky is fermented)

Single malt whiskey can control diabetes, reduce cancer risk, prevent heart disease, boost memory, it reduces stress, *boosts immune system*, lower LDL, *increase lifespan* and lower weight. I may add one tsp or tbsp to my coffee or drink 8oz in one week.

FOODS THAT ASSIST DIABETICS

Apples

Avocado

Barley (a lot more beneficial for diabetics than rice)

Beans

Berries

Bitter Melon (Sometimes I may take bitter melon pills for healthy blood sugar although I am not a diabetic.)

Broccoli

Flaxseeds (fights diabetes, cancer, heart disease)

Green tea, Black tea, Chamomile tea (Page 122)

Mushrooms

Oatmeal

Okra (Let okra water set overnight. Page 23, 92)

Spinach

Tomato

Turmeric (Turmeric milk is a blood purifier. See pg 64 Turmeric on pg 2 and 191 is for pain. Page 215 is great for nourishing the liver or fighting a **fatty liver**. Pg 63)

Eating a majority raw, low calorie, whole food diet consisting of mostly plant life is great and very beneficial for people with diabetes. Elevated blood glucose has been said to possibly normalize in about 2-3 weeks when one eliminates animal foods. Minimize starchy foods and natural sugars from fruit. Starchy foods require excess insulin to metabolize. If watching your fruit intake, the fruit itself has less sugar than store fruit juices. Eat fatty fish, peanut butter, legumes, nuts, eggs and protein shakes. They are high in protein and an increase in healthy fat helps with a sugar detox. Page 142

When I was first introduced to bitter melon, I was very excited. I knew that I had some great news to share with my newly diagnosed sister as well as many other people that have been diagnosed with diabetes. I know some people have already heard about this vegetable but there are many that are unaware of bitter melon. My sister has tried the pill form and the vegetable. The vegetable was to bitter for her but she is a fan of the pill. After taking the pill for awhile, she wondered if the pill was losing it's power. I suggested her cycling on and off the pill to see if anything improved. She agreed and so far, everything appears to be going well again.

Bitter melon is actually a member of the squash family. It resembles a cucumber with bumpy skin. When first picked, a bitter melon is yellow-green, but as it ripens, it turns to a yellow-orange color. As the fruit ripens, the flesh becomes tougher and more bitter. Bitter melon is used mostly in Asian and Indian recipes. This melon is generally cooked and consumed in the green stage. Bitter melon is typically stir-fried in Chinese cooking or used for soups. Bitter melon teas are also available. Bitter melon has been used for diabetes for many years. Gastrointestinal diseases, malaria, measles, certain cancers and chickenpox can also be fought with it.

Possible Bitter Melon Health Benefits

1. Bitter melon has *"insulin like"* polypeptide-p.

2. Bitter melon can possibly help in the treatment of Alzheimer's disease, prostate cancer, cholesterol and of course diabetes.

3. Boiled bitter melon extracts show antioxidant activities.

Bitter Melon Precautions

1. Bitter melon used short term is typically safe for healthy adults when consumed in moderation.

2. Possible bitter melon side effects include liver inflammation and spontaneous abortion. Pregnant women should avoid bitter melon.

3. The covering on the seed could possibly be toxic in children.

4. If uncertain, seek a professional doctor's advice.

Since buying the bitter melon tablets, my sister has ran across a plant based herb called Gymnema sylvestre. Gymnema sylvestre is an herb native to the tropical forest of southern and central India. Chewing the natural leaves can help suppresses the sensation and desire to eat many sweets. Gymnema sylvestre has been used in herbal medicine as a treatment for diabetes for many years. My sister has been using and enjoying the tablet forms of bitter melon and Gymnema sylvestre. She usually keeps one or both of them handy at all times.

Sugar, in all forms is a simple carbohydrate that the body converts into glucose and uses for energy. The effect sugar will have on your body and your overall health will depend on the type of sugar you are eating. Natural or refined. Natural sugars are found in fruit as fructose and in dairy products like milk and cheese as lactose. Refined sugar normally comes from sugar cane. Sugar is typically found as sucrose, which is the combination of glucose and fructose. As I mentioned in the publication *Your Health And Healing*, anything that ends in "ose" is usually a sugar. Once the sugar passes through the stomach and reaches the small intestine, it doesn't matter if it came from a candy bar or an apple, our body will use excess sugar according to how much sugar you already have in your blood. If you have a lot of sugar in your system, what you have left will turn into fat or glycogen for quick energy.

(I don't have a section on *beef liver* but it has been called a Super Food. It can aid diabetes and helped my **MS diagnosis**. Eat in moderation. Pg 151, #9.)

MULTIPLE SCLEROSIS

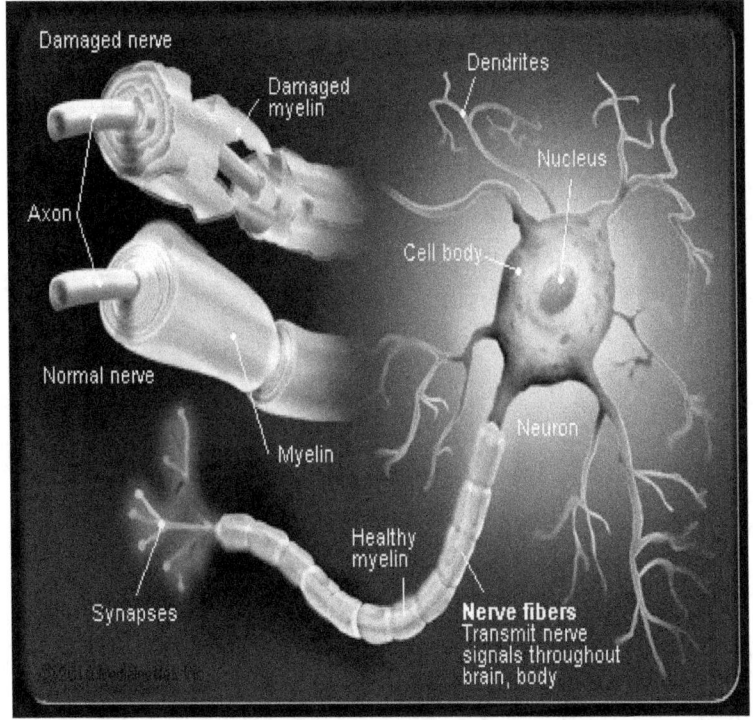

Last but certainly not least, let's discuss multiple sclerosis. This is the disease that decided to attack me. I have read some studies where they suggest that MS is hereditary and I have read some studies that suggest that it is not. I personally don't believe MS is hereditary. I say this because I am the only one on my father's side of the family and the only one on my mother's side of the family that has ever been diagnosed with MS. The fact I just shared is why my opinion stands that MS is not hereditary. Some families have habits that are shared by other family members. I believe influenced habits make MS appear hereditary if newer family members are also diagnosed. I think deficiencies + stress = MS.

Since writing *My MS Success,* you can say my diet has kinda evolved from the section titled "My Solution". My Solution is the chapter in *My MS Success* where I first explained what my method was that allowed me to achieve victory over MS. The method explained then, only covers what my known regime was during my first 2-3 years. The method I listed was not as simple to understand for readers as I wanted it to be. I basically just told the reader, *"These are all the foods I consumed on a regular basis to achieve my success".* This method of explaining was to broad and I don't think it was specific enough for the reader that may have been diagnosed with MS to easily apply and achieve the results they were seeking. The larger the variety of nourishment, the more difficult it will be to know which drink, meat, fruit or vegetable is providing the most healing. The explanation I currently share is basically the same, I just have more knowledge, a better understanding and the ability to explain the methods for my success so others can apply them to their lives. The breakdown of "My Solution" on fighting MS that I've included in this publication is broken down and explained more accurately. This time it is in regards to my more than 13 years of success I acquired and not the 2-3 years of success. I believe this latest explanation and plan of attack on MS will be the answer that many MS patients have been looking for. I want to be sure the reader absolutely understand my solution on fighting MS. (*Natural folate* **(B9)** absorbs at 50% **vs** *synthetic folate (folic acid)* at 85%. **Folic** is more heat stable.) Page 96

MULTIPLE SCLEROSIS

IT HAD TO HAPPEN

Early 2014 my battle with MS slowly went sour and it later intensified. I went from walking proud and standing strong to being nervous and skeptical. I became nervous because it was difficult to walk downstairs or upstairs. I couldn't move from room to room without some type of assistance. Falling to the left, to the right, backward or forward had all become normal and very scary to me. Imagine how I felt trying to step out of the shower, knowing I had to step head first to exit out. Falling down had basically become inevitable if I stood without any assistance. The assistance from my cane, walker or some other prop still did not guarantee total safety. I fell multiple times using my walker. My core and back had become very weak, they felt almost non-existent. If I fell backwards, my head would often snap back and bump the floor upon landing. While lying in the bed, many times I tested the accuracy of my kicks by kicking imaginary objects on the ceiling with my feet when I was healthy. I was now unable to accurately kick the imaginary objects on the ceiling with my feet. I could no longer snap my fingers with ease, definitely not with my left hand. I could not snap my fingers or make the snapping sounds at all. Cramps were recurring, fatigue had resurfaced and once again, I was not able to stand long periods at a time. "I had to crawl a lot." In my opinion, this flare up was definitely worse than my very first encounter with MS back when I was first diagnosed in 97. However, I believe that this most recent episode had to happen. It was going to allow me another opportunity to take my time and really focus on the task that was at hand. With all of the knowledge and experience I had acquired, my plan was to find a definitive answer to the success I had enjoyed for so long. I figured that I might have to suffer to achieve the goal I was seeking but I was perfectly Ok with that. I wanted and needed a clear route to optimal health not just for myself but for others that are suffering and seeking help. I began observing any positive or negative results from the specific food and liquids I was ingesting and I took notes. I knew God was in the plans and I knew that everything was going to be just fine. I made it my goal that after achieving victory and reclaiming my health again, I was going to put my results in print. Why did my health fail? "My MS Setback", Pg 36.

Excess Sugar Can Be Very Harmful

Based on my own experience and observations, excessive sugar (especially refined sugar) could be a very serious threat to MS patients. Sugar can be addictive and hard to resist. Excessive amounts can present very harmful and devastating effects on our health such as irritate your immune system, disrupt your digestive system and cause varied side effects that can seriously harm your body. Ahead are other instances where I was negatively affected by eating to much sugar. I had began **a new workout regime** of lifting weights and working out. My goal was to increase my strength and achieve a more muscular tone. I began to add a lot of pasta to my diet daily. My main objective was to allow my body to burn the carbohydrates in the pasta for energy and allow my body to easily use the protein I was consuming for muscle growth. After a few weeks, I began to observe slight complications walking and my foot would drag off and on. For those that do not know, a constant or an occasional foot drag is one of the main symptoms associated with MS. Not until my walk began to change, I had no idea that I had been consuming sugar in excess. Refined carbohydrates like macaroni, pasta, white flour, refined cereals, white rice and noodles can have the same effect on our body as refined sugar. My family has a history of diabetes so I consume sugar in moderation now. Again, excess sugar can be very harmful. (**Glucose:** #1 sugar for fuel, our brain, nerve cells etc. Page 25)

Aspartame & Multiple Sclerosis

Years ago, I heard that there was a possibility that the sweetener aspartame could be linked to causing multiple sclerosis. I do not believe that aspartame causes MS but I believe that it should be left alone by any MS patient. I feel this way because one day I was having a very bad headache, so I checked my dietary diary to study my recent regimen. I noticed bottled water with *added flavor* was a new addition to the list of my current liquids and foods. As I was reading the ingredients of the bottled water flavors, I noticed that one of them had aspartame listed 3rd in the ingredients. Anytime aspartame was listed 4th or below, bad headaches never followed. I came to the conclusion that if aspartame was listed 3rd in the ingredients or higher, I will just leave it alone because obviously that's to much aspartame for my system. I saw that aspartame can drastically trigger negative effects in a MS patient. After doing some research, I discovered aspartame could cause some serious problems so I stop consuming it. Pg 17, #5

Within the next 24 hrs, the headache was gone and after that episode, I never had that problem again.

My MS Setback (Just **1** cough drop has 3-4 g sugar.)

In the previous section titled "**It had to happen**", you can see how the devastating effects of to much sugar affected my health. This next situation, I had a hard time trying to figure out why my health was failing me. I was eating healthy and watching what I was consuming. I had recently purchased a new healthy product. I read the container correctly but the mistake I made, was failing to read it carefully. This product was made from a very nutritional and reputable fruit. I was so enthused to finally get my hands on this product that I bought a lot of the 12oz bottles. I was drinking about 3 a day. As my health began to fail I wondered what was wrong with my diet. It took me awhile but it finally dawned on me, I had negligently failed to read the sugar content in the product I was consuming per serving. The 12oz bottles I was consuming had 33 grams of sugar **per serving**. Each bottle had 3 servings. That's to much sugar for anyone to consume in the manner I was drinking them. Even my enzyme rich diet had little affect improving my health. Eat enzyme rich foods but avoid excess sugar intake. Improvements could began to show in a few days or it may take some time. Results will vary depending on each person. All the MS stories I shared with you in this chapter had solutions. The aspartame incident I mentioned earlier was the easiest/fastest MS problem I solved. I mentioned it for aspartame awareness purposes. Diet solutions that I used to fight MS and gain my health back from previous episodes are ahead.

My Solution

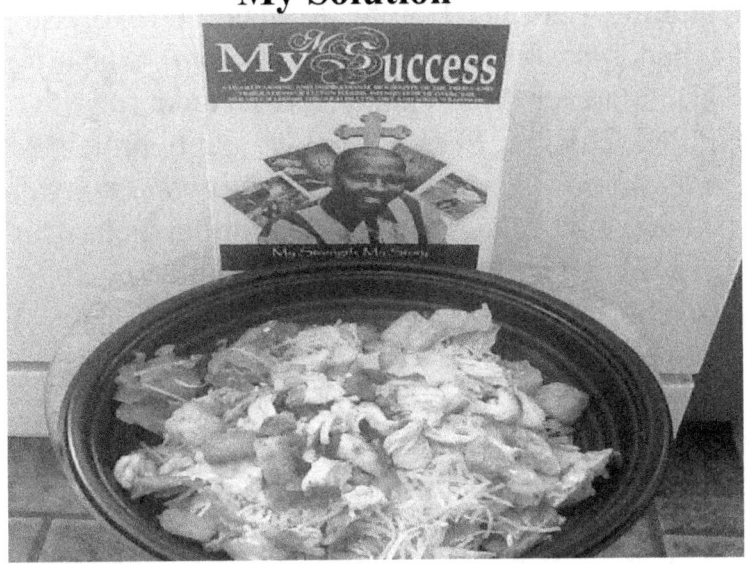

1. For 13 plus years and at least 3 times a week, I consumed a full sized salad. This is the #1 salad I used to stay healthy. It proved to be instrumental to my MS success and overall health. Due to the large amount of different foods I was consuming at that time, it was difficult trying to pinpoint which foods were actually benefiting me and which were not. The human body needs vital nutrients every day. The absence of just one could mean the difference in success or failure. I use vegetables that are *fresh daily* to assist in achieving this goal so this salad will be full of nutrients, oxygen and live enzymes so it can perform the healing process at it's best. I add chicken and cheese to my salads because they can provide the amino acids tyrosine and carnitine. They both assist in muscle movement and reflexes. Carnitine needs carbohydrates (most meals have it) to properly absorb and tyrosine needs vitamin C. (See page 174, 182 and 212 plus 89, 135 and 211.)

Romaine Lettuce: I prefer Romaine due to taste, the benefits (*pg 85*), Vitamin K (*pg 146*), silica (*pg 163*), folate, enzymes and it has *lactucin (*pg 86*).
Grilled Chicken Breast for 35g quality protein & *sphingolipids* (*see chicken pg 75 & protein pg 157*)
Cheese: I like *cheddar* or mixed for the dietary fat (*pg 141*), whey (*pg 206*) & sphingolipids (*pg 208*).
Bruschetta Topping (or Pico topping or tomatoes)
1 cup chopped plum tomatoes (*about 2 tomatoes*)
1/4 cup chopped red onion (*about 1/4th of an onion*)
2 tablespoons drained and chopped roasted red peppers (*packed in water*)
2 tablespoons sliced black olives, finely chopped
1 tablespoon chopped fresh basil
1/2 teaspoon chopped garlic
Guacamole many health benefits (*see pg 191*)
Mexican Ranch Dressing (nutrient absorption)
¼ cup mayonnaise
¼ cup sour cream
1 Tbs milk
2 tsp minced tomato
1½ tsp white vinegar
1 tsp minced canned jalapeño slices
1 tsp minced onion
¼ tsp dried parsley (*I use dried parsley in many recipes*)
¼ tsp Tabasco pepper sauce
1/8 tsp salt
1/8 tsp dried dill weed
1/8 tsp paprika
1/8 tsp cayenne pepper
1/8 tsp cumin
1/8 tsp chili powder

MULTIPLE SCLEROSIS

1 dash garlic powder
1 dash freshly-ground black pepper
1 cup shredded Cheddar-Jack cheese
Tortilla Chips (For the salt content. *See pg 160*)

2. Sub Sandwiches have been instrumental to my overall health as well. Lettuce, tomatoes, spinach, cucumbers, olives, onions, bell peppers, cheese, mustard, olive oil and chicken, turkey or steak are the toppings I prefer. Oregano or honey oat are the breads I prefer at the restaurant. (Oregano can be used for respiratory tract disorders such as coughs, asthma and bronchitis. It is used to treat spasms, heartburn, rheumatoid arthritis, menstrual cramps, headaches, urinary tract infections (UTI) and heart conditions.) Some restaurants may not add enough leafy green lettuce. If you have time, you can make a homemade sub. Eating vegetables that are *fresh daily* provide more *nutrition, oxygen* and *enzymes*.

3. Fish: I eat fish with broccoli and carbs like rice or bread often. I keep omega-3s and *fish collagen* in my diet regime. Our body absorbs *fish collagen* easier than *chicken collagen*. (The collagen/amino acids differ.) Unwanted ingredients will appear in certain *marine collagen (page 180)*. I believe eating fish often boost my speed and reflexes in sports as well as my gait after my MS diagnosis. (pg 80, 114)

4. Chicken (grilled/broiled): I eat chicken for the protein with pico or carbs like potatoes, pasta etc. This allows the *carnitine* to *absorb better.* (pg 212) I add chicken to stuffed potatoes too. I add cheese, chicken and butter to potatoes because I want extra *sphingolipid* content (*pg 208*). Dried basil, parsley or chives are used due to vitamin K (*pg 146*). When I buy cheese, I prefer the **1**st ingredient to be *whey*. **Steak & potatoes** is another one of my top meals. For best results, I use 100% natural potatoes.

5. Eggs, Oatmeal, OJ: Many times I eat two eggs along with oatmeal and orange juice for breakfast. I now eat eggs for the *sphingolipids* (*page208*). Iron found in oatmeal is important (*page 150*). OJ helps the iron absorb better. Drinking orange juice with oatmeal or *high carbohydrate food* with a *sensible amount of fat* helps fight *inflammation*. Eating non processed oatmeal while drinking orange juice can clean our arteries and help prevent heart attacks. At times I'll add two bacon slices for the fat (*page 141*) and *myelin forming* B1 (*page 156*). Bacon is the **2**nd highest source of **carnitine**. (*page 80, 123, 182, 212*)

6. Kellog's Total whole grain cereal has 100% DV of multiple vitamins and minerals. It has 100% DV of *myelin repairing* folic acid and *myelin forming* B1. I have ate 2 bowls a day on multiple occasions. I add almonds for extra nutrition. (*page 67 #11*)

7. Isopure is *oxygen rich*, it has 50% RDA of many vitamins, minerals, 50g of quality *whey* protein per serving and amino acids. In 2000, I began taking 2 scoops **2x** a day Mon-Fri. My health improved.

8. B12 boosts the *nervous system, myelin sheath,* DNA regulation etc. Sources: *mackerel, sardines, clams, fortified cereal, Total has 100%.* See B1, B3 pg 156. **Iron/Zinc:** *beef, clams* **p**76, *oyster, poultry*

I feel great when Isopure is in my system. I drink Isopure Mon-Fri, 2 times a day. I consume it after I exercise and many times on an **empty stomach**. I eat *folate* rich foods (*pg 96*) and I consume the #1 - #8 options listed often. These options work best for me after I fast (*pg 61*). The #1 salad provides the 4 essential food groups. I normally eat it 1-2 hrs after Isopure. This has helped me work and manage MS with great success for more than 13 years. (*pg 205*)

When a person begins eating, the stomach starts producing HCL (hydrochloric acid/stomach acid). HCL is necessary for proper digestion and immune health. Without it, food isn't digested correctly and that could cause a vitamin and mineral deficiency. Proteins wouldn't be broken down properly and a protein deficiency could develop. The body would need to rob protein from joint surfaces and move it to the areas where needed. Eat your protein food at the beginning of your meal since it needs HCL for proper digestion. The carbohydrates that make up a salad **require no HCL** for digestion, so it is fine to eat your salad last or with some protein. To avoid a risk of HCL production being lowered, **do not eat large amounts** of processed or fast foods, refined carbohydrates, refined sugars, antacids, ice water with meals, an unhealthy acidic diet or when upset. HCL production is slowed by stress, so relax while you're eating. Consume natural salt, live food, take quality multivitamins, chew your food thoroughly and increase your zinc. **Hot/warm:** coffee, ginger, green/black tea or warm lemon water will increase stomach acid production. See page 164 and 207.

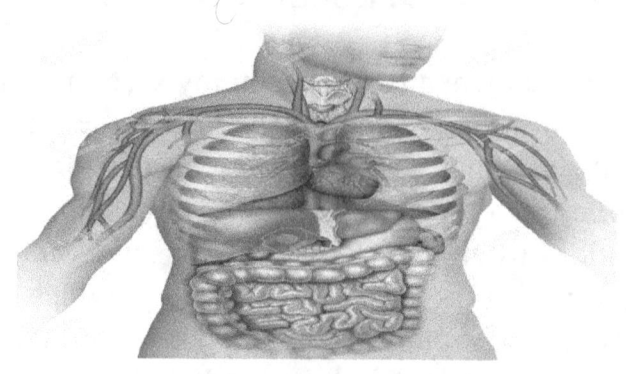

ORGANS

CLEAN ARTERIES

Eating foods that clean out the arteries will not only lead to improved cardiovascular health, it will improve digestion, aid in weight loss, ease joint pain and increase metabolism. Balanced nutrition increases our energy levels and alertness through greater circulation of oxygen throughout the body and to the brain. Continuing to eat heart healthy foods that are rich in fiber and antioxidants, low in cholesterol and low in bad fats, will ensure long-term cardiac health. Eating foods that clean your arteries will have an effect on your blood pressure. Always consult with your doctor before changing your diet. If you desire better circulation and blood flow in you arteries, the following foods can assist you.

1. Apples
2. Garlic
3. Garbanzo beans

4. Grapefruit
5. Green/Black Tea
6. Olive oil
7. Salmon: Inhibits coronary artery calcification, it can reduce the oxidation of cholesterol & stimulate the production of nitric oxide in the lining of blood vessels.
8. Spinach
9. Swiss Chard
10. Tomatoes: The Lycopene aid in clean arteries.
11. Beets: Cleans blood and system, nature's viagra. Beets contain oxalic acid. Most people's bodies can process oxalic acid but if it can't, kidney stones can form. Eat beets in moderation, not in excess.

CLEAN COLON

The last five feet of our digestive system/tract is the colon. The colon is your large intestine that is often referred to as the large bowel. It is the part of the intestine from the cecum to rectum. The colon helps clear our system of toxins, fecal matter and waste. The most critical function of the colon is to absorb the water, minerals, vitamins and to prepare and store fecal waste prior to elimination. There is a very delicate balance of bacteria in our colon and it assists our colon in natural functioning. Normal colon functioning can become inhibited and off track if certain bacteria is not properly balanced. Proper bacteria in the intestinal tract helps build a *stronger immune system*. A strong immune system is what is needed for assimilation of fats, proteins, amino acids, carbohydrates and vitamins such as Vitamin K. (K aids in proper blood clotting)

When we consume our food, the food ingested should not set in our body for long periods at a time. The food we ingest should normally be ready to exit our bodies in less than twenty-four hours. If your bowel movements are not regular, the waste products and toxins are accumulating and that can compromise your health. The waste will begin to decay and leave residue of fecal matter behind. Prolonged food in the bowels create a disease-friendly environment in the colon. The longer the food lingers in our colon, the more it allows toxins a chance to penetrate the bowel wall and pass to the blood system. This problem could later spread throughout the body causing a weakened *immune system*. A weakened *immune system* can lead to a faster development of many major diseases such as cancer, heart disease, diabetes and other unwanted ailments. With one bowel movement per day, it is still possible to have an estimated amount of about three meals worth of waste matter accumulated in your colon. Elimination of fecal matter becomes incomplete and waste can remain in the intestines. Less than three bowel movements a week may indicate constipation and more than three watery stools a day could indicate diarrhea. When your colon is not functioning properly, waste can leak into your bloodstream. If this happens, it is known as "*auto-intoxification*". Bowel movements should be soft and easy to pass, not hard and difficult.

Two causes of bowel malfunction are insufficient water intake and lack of physical exercise but the main cause of bowel malfunction revolves around malnutrition. Most people do not consume enough nourishing foods to supply the muscles and tissues of the bowel with the nutrients needed. The result is the bowel begins to deteriorate and and lose it's muscle tone. The body needs enough roughage or fiber to push the wastes through the colon. Keep in mind that if a person has lived a lifetime of poor eating habits, immense damage to the colon could have occurred to a point where even the best and correct diet may take awhile to render good results.

Why Is Your Colon Not Functioning 100%?

Stress, drugs and chemicals can all help lead to an irritated and poor functioning bowel. Some of the main foods to avoid eating **large amounts** of that can harm and irritate the colon are animal products (red meat, pork), salt, sugar and flour. So, in other words, a "Bad Diet". These foods have no life and will provide no energy to the digestive system. The quality of the food you eat will impact your overall health.

The human body goes through great lengths to protect itself from danger. If the colon is irritated by unhealthy foods we consume, it will produce a mucus plaque to protect itself. The plaque covers our digestive tract and helps prevent the body from absorbing dangerous toxins into the bloodstream. Ironically the plaque is produced using the very same unhealthy foods that was just consumed. The more food you continue to eat that's unhealthy, the thicker the plaque becomes and the mucus plaque then binds with food residue from the previous accumulated foods. The plaque becomes hardened and binds to the colon walls. The first goal of the mucus plaque was for it to block dangerous toxins from entering your blood system. With continuous and constant unhealthy eating, it begins blocking important vitamins and minerals from entering as well. I read part of one medical examiner's autopsy report where he examined the colon of a deceased male. He stated that the colon had so much plaque buildup as well as so many impurities that it would be difficult to cut the colon with a knife.

Symptoms associated with an unhealthy colon include constipation, fatigue, headache, spots, poor skin, muscle/joint aches, stomach pain, digestive problems, weight gain, premature aging, gas, poor eyesight, hair loss, memory loss, chronic fatigue, diarrhea, depression, emotional instability, bloating and much more. Food trapped inside the colon can easily breed bacteria and harmful parasites. It has been estimated that around 150 million people in America have intestinal parasite infestation. There are more than 300 parasite varieties that can live in the human body. Many people are walking around with parasites in their body right now but they are totally unaware.

Methods That Can Help Clean Your Colon

There are several methods that you can use to cleanse your colon. Colon hydrotherapy, laxatives, *colonic fasting* regime and nutritional supplement aids are some of the most popular methods. I had a colon hydrotherapy cleanse session with water and abdominal massage performed before. The purpose of a hydrotherapy cleanse is to remove toxins from the fat, muscle, blood and internal organs that have accumulated over a period of years due to poor/unhealthy eating. The water and the massage helped break up the unwanted matter within the small and large intestines with excellent results. This will help prevent disease. The body's immune system is the first line of defense against almost all infections and diseases. If your body has a strong immune system you will be less prone to infection. When you have a cleanse performed you loosen, break up and flush out the accumulated waste and poison. Clean organs result in good health and the colon is the best place to begin with. It would be next to impossible to restore optimal health with a filthy, unclean colon.

People can achieve great benefits from a colon hydrotherapy when it is done in conjunction with fluids, exercise and diet. Other successful methods to remove waste from the walls of your stomach, small intestine and colon are listed ahead.

1. Chew your food thoroughly.

2. Eat high volumes of fresh fruit and vegetables.

3. Vanilla bean helps optimize digestive function.

4. A 2-3 day "no food fast" can *reboot the immune system*. **Fasting** is a profitable colon cleanse. Pg 61

5. Hydrate, dissolve, disinfect and help soothe your intestinal tissue with plenty of water and healthy fluids. Warm water flushes toxins better than cold.

6. Fiber has the capacity to extract many feet of mucus from the intestinal walls in a short period of time. Fruits are solvents in the system and acid fruits are the strongest. 35 - 40 grams is good.

(A healthy diet and fasting regime can end cleanses.)

Benefits 2 Expect From A Colon Hydrotherapy Cleanse Are:

1. Weight loss

2. Clearer skin

3. Increased energy levels

4. Improved concentration

5. Overall healthful feeling

6. Regular bowel movements

7. Better mental health and memory

8. Reduced gas and food sensitivities

9. Better absorption of vitamins and minerals from foods (Replenish your electrolytes and probiotics.)

Himalayan/Sea Salt Water Cleanse (Low cost)
2 level teaspoons, non-iodized Pink/sea salt (Never use table salt, Dead sea salt or Epsom salt)

1 quart (32 oz) purified water (Lukewarm)
(16 oz has been reasonable for some.)

Instructions:

1. Put 2 teaspoons of sea salt into 32 oz/quart jar.

2. Pour in warm water and stir.

3. Drink entire 32 oz of saltwater first thing in the morning on empty stomach. Drink it kinda quickly. (8oz warm water, with 2 **tsp salt**, on **empty** stomach is great but it is not the same as a hydrotherapy cleanse.)

4. Lie on your right side for 30 minutes to help the saltwater reach the lower right hand side of the stomach, where the opening to the small intestine is located. Gently massage your stomach off and on during this process.

5. After 30 minutes, you are free to move about as you wish. Be sure to remain near a restroom. The saltwater stimulates contractions in your stomach that propel the sea salt solution through your digestive system. For me, 35 minutes later it was time to expel but individual results may vary. Some people may need to expel multiple times. I only needed to expel once. The bowel movement may be intense diarrhea but that is perfectly normal. The saltwater quickly cleanses your entire digestive tract. If you develop the urge to pass gas, be sure you are on the toilet if you decide to until you are certain that the expel process is complete. Any minor discomfort or paranoia you may have during this process should improve quickly after the cleanse. An hour after the first time you expel should be enough time were the body is back to normal and the restroom does not have to be your best friend anymore. I did not vomit or even come close but vomiting is normal for a select few.

BEST FIBER RICH FOODS TO CLEAN THE COLON AND PUSH FOOD THROUGH

Apples 4.4g, Almonds 3g quarter cup, Artichokes 10.3g cup, Avocado 2g 2tbs, Barley, Citrus Fruit

Black Beans 15g cup, Broccoli 5.1g cup, Brown Rice 3.5g cup, Corn 2g ½ cup, Dark Leafy Greens

Edamame Beans 9g half cup, Garbanzo/Chick Peas, Garlic, Kidney Beans, Lentils 15.6 cup,

Oatmeal, Peas 16.3g cup, Unpeeled Pears 5.5g, Apple Cider Vinegar, Milk, Whole Wheat Bread

Whole Wheat Pasta, White Beans, Raspberries 1/3 of fiber needs cup, Water (move fiber and waste out)

*Fiber can lower blood sugar, cut cholesterol and help prevent colon cancer. If you peel or remove the peeling from an apple or from a pear, you are throwing away beneficial phytochemicals (**natural bioactive compounds that are found in fruits and vegetables that work with vitamins, minerals and fiber to promote good health**) and fiber. Excessive intake of fiber can decrease the body's absorption of iron and other important minerals.*

Heal colon: applesauce, bananas, oatmeal, poultry, fish, eggs, mashed potato, canned fruit, rice, cereal
IBD Trigger foods: fried/fatty foods, spicy foods, red meat, alcohol, sweets, caffeine, high fiber food, beans, nuts, seeds, creamy sauces, candy, soda

HEALTHY HEART

Exercise is one of the most important factors in healthy heart health. Please do not neglect to do it. The heart needs the workout. I am pretty sure that you have a general idea on what type foods that are not very heart healthy. Foods such as fatty meats, butter, gravy, fried foods, cakes, pies and fast food in general can all cause problems for the heart over time. If you know which foods to avoid, you also need to know which foods are best for your heart. You can start fighting heart disease by adding these foods to your diet. Some great, heart-healthy foods are ahead. (**Menhaden:** #1 heart health fish, Page 53)

1. Salmon (softgels are fine, specially for **Menhaden**)

Salmon is loaded with antioxidants and omega-3 fatty acids. Salmon can help reduce blood pressure and prevent blood clotting. Wild salmon has been said to provide more health benefits than their farm raised coequal. (**Menhaden** is to bony & oily to eat.)

2. Olives/Olive oil

3. Oatmeal

4. Flaxseed

Flaxseed is one of the best whole grains to use for keeping your heart in great shape.

5. Nuts

6. Beans

7. Dark green vegetables, Spinach, Okra (**vitamin k** is found in green vegetables, vitamin **K1** can be found in fermented vegetables and foods.) See page 146, 206

8. Avocados, beets, purple grapes

9. Blueberries, strawberries, raspberries: Berries in general are great *anti-inflammatory* foods that can help reduce the risk of heart disease.

Heart Attack Risk Symptoms

1. Dizziness

2. Lack of appetite

3. Fatigue and feeling tired all the time may be a symptom of heart failure.

4. Chest discomfort. Pain in the chest is the classic No.1 symptom of heart attack.

5. Anxiety. Heart attack can cause intense anxiety or a fear of death in heart attack survivors.

6. Persistent coughing, wheezing or throwing up bloody phlegm can be a symptom of heart failure.

7. Pain in the chest, shoulders, arms, back, neck, abdomen, elbows or jaw. The pain could come and go periodically.

8. Shortness of breath normally accompanies chest discomfort but it can also occur with or without chest discomfort.

9. Rapid and irregular pulse along with weakness, dizziness or shortness of breath can be evidence of a heart attack, heart failure, or arrhythmias. If one leaves arrhythmias untreated it can lead to stroke, heart failure or sudden death.

10. Weight Gain

11. Unexplained weakness

12. Abdomen, feet or ankle swelling

13. Breaking out in cold sweat, sweating profusely like you have just worked out

Avoid The Following For A Healthier Heart

A. Smoking
B. Heavy drinking
C. Eating high-fat foods

Foods To Avoid Heart Burn

After experiencing the worst, most uncomfortable heartburn I had ever experienced (periodically) for more than two weeks, it was time to study and try to figure out what was happening. What had I been ingesting? The following 1-10 list will show you some "high risk heart burn causing items" to avoid if you are experiencing heartburn. If a star is next to it, that just means that I myself was consuming that very particular item during the "more than two week uncomfortable heart burn" time frame I just mentioned. I used the baking soda remedy found under *Foods That Neutralize Heart Burn* (Page 55 #4). Heart burn was nullified almost instantly. The **Wild Caught Menhaden** has DHA, EPA and the rare, heart healthy, superior omega-3;**DPA**. Page 80

Calcium + vitamin D can fight cancer, diabetes & HBP. Our **heart**, *strong bones*, *muscles* and *nerves* all *need calcium* to function properly. Page 74, 181

1. Alcohol* (Was trying to add the mineral *silica* in my system to help flush out any harmful *aluminum* that was potentially in my body. I am not a drinker so drinking beer definitely did not last long.)

2. Caffeine*

3. Types of aspirin

4. Ibuprofen*
   Motrin
   Advil
   Nuprin

5. Naproxen
   Naprosyn
   Aleve)

6. Carbonated beverages

7. Acidic juices
   Grapefruit*
   Orange*
   Pineapple*

8. Acidic foods
   Tomatoes*
   Grapefruit*
   Oranges*

9. Chocolate*

10. Smoking

Foods That Neutralize Heart Burn

On pg 53, I shared some foods and juice you may want to stay away from to avoid heartburn. Ahead you will find some effective foods and juice to help neutralize heart burn.

1. Ginger Tea

2. Aloe Vera Juice (High doses of Aloe can cause diarrhea, a vitamin and mineral imbalance and/or abdominal pain. Drink Aloe Vera in moderation.)

3. Cabbage juice (For best results, drink cabbage juice in the morning on an empty stomach.)

4. Baking Soda (Half a tbsp dissolved in a glass of water is recommended. It's OK to use a little more. I used one tbsp.)

5. Apple Cider Vinegar (Two tbsp of ACV mixed in half cup of water. If ACV continues to bring no relief from heartburn, you may have to much acid built up in your system instead of not enough. At this point discontinue the use of ACV for fighting heart burn.)

Help And Tips On Fighting Heart Burn

A few other notes and tips to help fight heartburn are to increase your fiber, eat small portions, chew your food slowly and avoid eating any after dinner mints.

Selenium: heart protector, may fight MS (Page 211)

Proper consumption of selenium in your diet can lower heart disease. Selenium can reduce oxidation of cholesterol and stop blood clots from forming. Selenium can be found in the following foods.

1. Brazil nuts (Eat **only a few servings** a week.)

2. Fish (tuna, salmon, sardines, flounder, halibut)

3. Meat (beef, lamb, steak, liver, pork)

4. Eggs (To many can lower selenium absorption.)

5. Poultry (chicken breast, turkey)

6. Cheese (cheddar, Gouda, govt, hoop, Parmesan)

7. Mushrooms (white button, portobello, shiitake)

8. Shellfish (clams, mussel, oyster, lobster, shrimp)

9. Seeds (sunflower, Chia, sesame, pumpkin, flax)

10. Whole Grains (wheat germ, barley, brown rice, oats, oatmeal)

Low absorption: alcohol, coffee, smoking,white rice
Deficit: fatigue, hair loss, brain fog, a weak immunity

Krill Oil (Krill are small, shrimp like crustaceans.)
Krill oil costs more than fish oil, supplies omega-3 and astaxanthin. It can reduce joint pain, increase HDL and decrease LDL cholesterol better than fish oils. It is also more absorbable. **Astaxanthin** gives salmon it's reddish color. It cleans up our cells, it fights fatigue, supports eye health, it can keep our skin looking younger and it acts as a sunscreen.
Astaxanthin sources: Wild Pacific & Sockeye salmon

HOW CAN WATER HELP YOUR HEART

Drinking water on an empty stomach works in the treatment of the following ailments: TB, headache, body aches, heart system, accelerated heart beat, epilepsy, blood fat, bronchitis, asthma, meningitis, kidney disease and urinary tract, vomiting, piles, gastritis, diarrhea, diabetes, constipation, all eye diseases, diseases of the uterus, diseases of the ear, nose and throat as well as menstrual disorders.

"Heart Help" Water Treatment Method:
1. When you wake up in the morning & before you brush your teeth, drink 22oz of water. If you go by ml, that is 4 times 160ml of water (640ml).
2. Brush your teeth but do not eat and do not drink in the next 45 minutes.
3. After 45 minutes you can eat and drink normally again.
4. After your breakfast, lunch and dinner do not eat or drink anything for two hours.
5. If the person is older, sickly or if they can't drink 22oz/4 times 160ml of water on an empty stomach, they can start off by drinking as much as possible. They can increase their water intake each day until they reach the required 22oz or 4 times 160ml.
6. This method can cure different diseases & those who are healthy will enjoy the energy that is given to them from the water.
7. How many days are required for this treatment?
A. High blood pressure – 30 days
B. For gastritis – 10 days

C. Diabetes – 30 days
D. For constipation – 10 days
E. TB – 90 days

Some believe this method of drinking water on an empty stomach should be applied throughout life. The goal is to stay alive, healthy and full of energy.

Note: If fighting arthritis, this method might only last three days in the first week. Take a week off, then re-start applying it again daily. This treatment has no bad side effects except the need to go to the restroom often. Drink water and please stay active.

Other common facts about water consumption.

1. Two glasses of water after you wake up in the morning helps activate your internal organs.

2. One glass of water 30 min before you eat will help with digestion.

3. One glass before taking a shower or bath could help lower blood pressure.

4. One glass before you go to bed could help avoid a stroke or heart attack.

MYOGLOBIN: Diving mammals such as seals & whales can remain underwater for long periods at a time due to the *high myoglobin* in their muscles. I eat *myoglobin rich* foods often. I believe the vital *oxygen* and *iron* in them fight MS. Page 123,180

KIDNEYS

Our kidneys remove excess organic molecules from the blood, which allows the removal of waste products of metabolism. They are essential to the urinary system and they regulate electrolytes. Our kidneys maintenance the acid base balance and by maintaining the salt and water balance, they aid in the regulation of blood pressure. Kidneys serve the body as a natural filter of the blood and removes water-soluble wastes which are then diverted to the bladder. After urine is formed, the kidneys excrete wastes such as urea and ammonium. Kidneys are responsible for the re-absorption of water, glucose and amino acids. Our kidneys are very important organs and these are just some of the actions they perform to help our bodies keep working properly.

Kidney disease is commonly linked to people that suffer from diabetes, heart disease and high blood pressure. Obesity, autoimmune diseases, urinary tract infections and other infections can contribute to the risk of developing kidney disease. People over the age of 60 are more prone to developing kidney disease. Monitoring your blood pressure, cholesterol, blood glucose levels and not smoking are excellent decisions to good kidney health and kidney disease prevention. Be advised that kidney stones can develop when to many minerals build up in your urine. To help avoid mineral build up, eat a diet rich in fruits, vegetables and foods that are very low in salt. Exercising and drinking lots of water throughout the day is also beneficial to the kidneys. **Water is the best choice** but you can also drink fruit juices, ginger ale or tea. If your urine is light colored when you use the bathroom, then you know that you are drinking enough healthy fluids. Limit your caffeinated drinks to one to two cups a day if you enjoy them. Caffeinated beverages will help make you become dehydrated if not careful.

Grapes, cranberries, blueberries, fennel, onions, celery, beets, spinach, string beans and asparagus are some fruits and vegetables that can improve your kidney function. However if you are suffering from kidney disease, make sure that the fruits and vegetables you consume are low in potassium. If your potassium level gets to high, you could be at a greater risk of suffering from a heart attack or stroke. Apples, beans, peppers, zucchini, eggplant, rice, pears, peas, peppers, corn and pasta are low potassium foods.

The kidneys play a major role in the production of red blood cells. Without properly functioning kidneys, your red blood cell count could easily become low. As a result, you may feel fatigued and your energy levels could suffer. Low iron could possibly be the case if you were diagnosed with chronic kidney disease. Eating iron-rich foods can help solve this problem. You will find some iron rich foods in the section titled "Iron" located in the NOTES chapter found on page 150.

Excellent Kidney Friendly Foods

1. Apples

2. Blueberries

3. Cabbage

4. Cauliflower

5. Cherries

6. Cranberries

7. Egg Whites

8. Fish (salmon, cod, halibut and tuna are best)

9. Garlic

10. Green Leaf Lettuce

11. Olive Oil

12. Onions

13. Raspberries

14. Red Bell Pepper (#1 choice)

15. Red Grapes

16. Strawberries

FASTING REGIME (**True** fasting forbids calories.)

Fasting benefits the whole body. I aim for 7 days, 12 hrs each (12am to 12pm or from 6am to 6am). **If I need** something to eat, I'll eat a few vegetables and/or fruit. I use this time for prayer and claiming my healing. Fasting lets our organs rest. Page 11

LIVER (The liver & kidney help produce **carnitine.**)

Our liver is a very important and crucial organ in our body. Without a healthy liver, the tissues of our bodies would quickly die from lack of energy and nutrients. The liver has an astonishing capacity for regeneration of dead or damaged tissues. The liver makes proteins that are vital for blood clotting and other functions. (Our only organ that regenerates.)

The liver performs functions that are related to digestion, metabolism, immunity and the storage of nutrients within the body. The liver's main job is to filter the blood coming from the digestive tract before passing it to the rest of the body. The liver also detoxifies chemicals and metabolizes drugs.

When we consume fried foods, processed foods, overeat or are exposed to stress and environmental pollutants our liver becomes overworked and can't properly process toxins and fat. There are a variety of foods like oatmeal that can nourish and cleanse the liver naturally. Premier liver cleansers have a *.

1. Apple* (green apple fight fatty liver better than red)

2. Asparagus

3. Avocado

4. Beets* (beetroot juice)

5. Berries (blueberries, raspberries, cranberries etc)

6. Coffee* (a top pick, drink moderately, limit sugar)

7. Cruciferous vegetables*, carrots, bell peppers

8. Garlic*

9. Grains (Alternative) - Alternative grains come from plants that are not related to the Grass family. They're not actually grains but are used like grains. Ex: (quinoa, millet, brown rice, buckwheat, amaranth)

10. Grapefruit

11. Grapes (Red and purple grapes are top choices.)

*Fight fatty liver: beans, coconut oil, seaweed, stevia, #1, #7, #18, soy (limit sodium, omit added sugar)Pg 27

12. Green Tea (also chamomile, ginger, peppermint)

13. Lemon*, Lime

14. Nuts (especially almonds and walnuts)

15. Olive Oil (unsaturated fats)

16. Papaya (best eaten 4-5 hours after a meal)

17. Protein (chicken, eggs*, fatty fish*, clean protein)

18. Turmeric*(Drink turmeric milk before bed. Pg 64)

19. Watermelon

PROSTATE

Prostate cancer is a common type of cancer found in men. Males 40 years of age or older may want to start early taking the necessary steps to prostate cancer prevention. An examination by a physician may be a wise choice. If treated at an early stage, it is highly curable and it has a high rate of recovery. Pay attention to the foods you consume. There are certain foods that can help protect, strengthen and aid your prostate health. They are listed ahead.

1. Omega-3 rich fish

2. Broccoli, cabbage, cauliflower

3. Nuts, seeds, wheat germ and whole grains due to their Vitamin E content

4. Tomatoes and red grapefruit can aid the prostate due to the lycopene. Lycopene is discussed more in detail on page 102 in regards to tomatoes.

5. Water and healthy liquids

6. Brazil nuts, seafood, some meats, fish, wheat bran, wheat germ, oats and brown rice all help the prostate due to their selenium content. Selenium is a powerful antioxidant (see *selenium* page 56).

7. *Avoid excess red and processed meats, caffeine filled drinks, spicy foods, high fat dairy, sugar, soy products and alcohol. Consume in **moderation**.

Broccoli and tomatoes both fight prostate cancer but *as a team* they can assist in *preventing* prostate cancer and possibly *shrink existing* prostate cancer tumors (*pg 70*). Turmeric/milk (½ tsp turmeric and milk) fights prostate cancer, diabetes, aids liver etc.

Spleen: eat **hot**, healthy food/drinks, not processed

Adrenal Glands

Adrenal glands modulate the functioning of every organ, tissue and gland in our body. They help our body deal with stress, has effects on how we think and feel. They are located on top of each kidney. I have sources that can strengthen the adrenal glands like **yams, licorice, celery** and **mushrooms** ahead.

Vitamin B: Pantothenic acid, beef, tuna, turkey,oats bananas, potatoes, avocados, Brazil nuts

Vitamin C: berries, broccoli, citrus fruits, peaches Brussels sprouts, mangoes, tomatoes, spring greens

Amino L-tyrosine: chicken, eggs, salmon, seaweed, cheese crystals (**tyrosine** or **calcium lactate**), oats

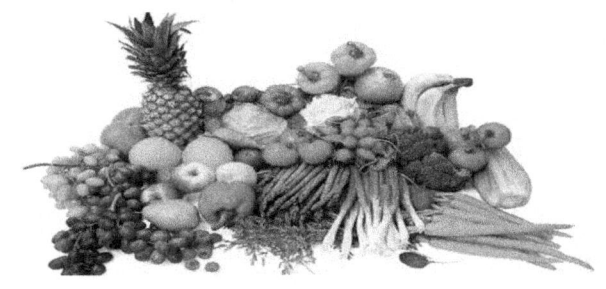

FOODS

When it comes to this chapter, please understand that the foods I have listed are not the only foods I consume. Some people think I am very limited as to what foods I eat. No!!! On occasions I eat fried foods, hamburgers, hot dogs, pizza and other foods that are not considered a healthy choice, just not consistently. I tell people all the time, *"I eat what I want to eat when I want to eat it. I let my healthy eating outweigh my unhealthy eating by a large margin."* The foods in this chapter are the foods I ate most during my most recent MS episode. These foods are loaded with healthy benefits that will give your body the nutrition it needs. *Eat starches/ carbs with veg but **eat fruit alone**. Studies find that chewing your food entirely results in better vitamin and mineral nutrient absorption. Try to consume a 20% acidity to 80% alkaline food ratio each day.*

ALMONDS

There are many health benefits that almonds can provide. Almonds have been used for relief from respiratory disorders, coughs, anemia, impotency, constipation and other important health problems. Almonds help the body absorb fat soluble vitamins due to it's healthy fat content. Some of the benefits almonds can provide you with are listed ahead.

1. Lower bad cholesterol

2. Help build strong bones and teeth

3. Almonds can *nourish the immune system.*

4. Almonds can help provide good brain function.

5. The potassium present in almonds help regulate blood pressure.

6. Good for the heart, can protect artery walls from damage, extra plaque and reduce heart attack risk.

7. Almonds have two very important fatty acids, *linoleic* and *linolenic acids.* These two fatty acids can *help reduce inflammation in the body.*

8. Almonds can help manage the absorption and processing of glucose, making the entire process so much smoother, safer and it offers protection from the dangerous spikes in blood sugar. Diabetics will occasionally suffer from a sugar spike following a large meal if the meal has an unexpected high level of sugar in it.

9. Almonds help alkalize the body and are the only nut that carries proteins that are alkaline forming. If your body is lacking alkalinity and is acidic, you could end up with osteoporosis, low energy, weight gain and/or a poor *immune function.*

10. Almonds improve the flow of food through the colon, which helps prevent build-up of waste and possible colon cancer. Fiber in almonds help with consistent bowel movements, elimination of toxins in the colon and can help in weight loss. They offer more iron, magnesium, E & good fat than peanuts.

11. At times I add almonds and/or almond milk to my Total cereal. More nutrition, better absorption.

12. The presence of manganese, copper and the B vitamin riboflavin can assist in energy production and metabolic rate.

13. Almond milk has been added to some soaps due to the almond's well established reputation for improving the complexion of our skin.

14. Almonds contain *folate* (natural form of *folic acid*). It is very beneficial for pregnant mothers.

Note: Avoid eating almonds if you have kidney or gallbladder problems.

APPLES (Any form will promote *colon cleansing.*)
After my MS diagnosis in the later 90s, I began to eat fresh apples or cooked apples with **cinnamon** a lot (*pg 192*). I began eating apples because I like them. I never knew how healthy apples were until I began to closely study their nutritional value. After suffering a MS setback in 2014, I began to eat a lot of cinnamon and apples again. Raw apples provide enzymes but even when cooked they still provide important healthy prebiotics (*see pg 206*). Unlike probiotics, cooking will not cause a significant loss in apple prebiotic fibers. Health benefits you can obtain by consuming apples are found ahead.

1. Help prevent cataracts
2. Help prevent gallstones
3. Help avoid hemorrhoids
4. *Boost immune system* (especially red apples)
5. Help eliminate constipation and/or diarrhea
6. Reduce cholesterol and strengthen the heart

7. Reduce the risk of *Type 2 Diabetes*

8. Control your weight, *bolster testosterone levels*

9. Detoxify your liver, protects against *Alzheimer's* and *Parkinson's disease, increase your nitric oxide*

10. Assist in fighting *pancreatic cancer.* An apple's high fiber content can reduce *colorectal* cancer and the peeling can help fight cancer cells in the colon, liver and breast. Ingest *applesauce, cider, juice* etc.

BANANAS

The banana has more vitamins and nutrients than an apple. A banana has about two times as many carbohydrates, five times as much Vitamin A and iron and close to three times as much phosphorus as an apple. If you are seeking energy then look no further. Eating two bananas can provide you with enough energy to exercise or workout for about an hour and a half. The energy a banana provides can give you a level of energy that will last longer than caffeine or sweets minus the infamous crash that is often caused by caffeine. On #16, I mentioned how bananas can also help give people suffering from anemia the iron their body may need. As healthy and beneficial as bananas are, eating a diet with to many bananas is not a wise idea. Doing so can be harmful to your health. Add variety. Occasionally I blend a banana with kefir and sometimes honey for an *enzyme rich* treat. Bananas help in many ways.

1. Protect against cramps

2. Help overcome depression

3. Pack an energy punch and sustain blood sugar

4. Aid digestion

5. Reduce swelling

6. Aid in weight loss

7. High in antioxidants

8. Lower blood pressure

9. Relieve stomach ulcers

10. Help stabilize blood sugar

11. Help prevent kidney cancer

12. Assist in absorbing nutrients

13. *Strengthen the nervous system*

14. Help normalize bowel motility

15. Protect against Type 2 Diabetes

16. Strengthen blood and relieve anemia

17. Protect against heart attack and stroke

18. Reduce nausea from morning sickness

19. Help restore lost electrolytes after diarrhea

20. Help with the production of white blood cells

21. Help make you more alert and increase libido

22. Protects the eyes against macular degeneration

23. Improve her mood and reduce PMS symptoms

24. Provide relief from acid reflux, heartburn and GERD

25. Can counteract calcium loss from urination and assist in building stronger bones.

26. Lower the body temperature during fever on a hot day
27. Speed recovery from the effects of smoking withdrawal
28. Eat fruit, nuts, seeds or eggs **alone**. Pg 151, #14

BROCCOLI

Broccoli is yet another important vegetable that I consumed during my 2014 MS battle. I had a lot of discomfort in my left arm daily for several months. The discomfort was more intense at night while trying to sleep than it was in the daytime. I did not go to the doctor because I assumed that perhaps it was arthritis. After I began to eat steamed Broccoli on a regular basis, the discomfort/arthritis I had in my left arm disappeared. It took less than a week for the positive effects to be noticed. On 9-29-14 my mother told me arthritis was bothering her arm. The discomfort in my mom's arm had bothered her longer than the discomfort I had. I asked her to try the same method I used. On 10-1-14 the arthritis in her arm was basically non-existent.

Broccoli is a super food and it is packed with a lot of tremendous health benefits. This important vegetable can be eaten raw or cooked. It is best to either steam or eat Broccoli raw to preserve it's nutrients. Broccoli has a plethora of carbohydrates, calcium, chromium, vitamin A, iron, vitamin C and it has a small amount of protein. *Both broccoli and tomatoes fight prostate cancer but if they are eaten together they can shrink prostate cancer tumors.*

Broccoli contains important phytochemicals and antioxidants. Both help fight various illnesses and infections. Broccoli can also help *clean our colon*. Many benefits broccoli can provide are ahead.

1. Anti-cancer properties
Against colon, prostate, cervical, breast and lung cancer

2. Anti aging properties
Broccoli has anti aging properties that can reverse the effect of the aging process.

3. Aid digestion
Broccoli is rich in fiber, which helps with digestion and works at dealing with or even preventing constipation

4. Acts as a detoxifier
The presence of vitamin C, certain amino acids and sulfur make broccoli a great detoxifier. Read # 8.

5. Control Diabetes
Broccoli is rich in chromium. Chromium is known to help regulate insulin and control diabetes.

6. Improve immune system

7. Maintain healthy eyesight
Broccoli is a good source of vitamin A. Vitamin A is needed to form retinal, that is the light-absorbing molecule that is essential for both low-light and color vision. Research has suggested that the beta-carotene in broccoli can protect the eyes against macular degeneration and prevent cataract.

8. Protect against UV radiation (help repair skin damage) A cup of Broccoli has as much Vitamin C as an orange. Steaming it will save many nutrients.

9. Weight Loss

10. Strengthen bones and prevent osteoporosis
Broccoli contains high levels of both calcium and vitamin K.

11. Prevent anemia
The Iron and folic acid found in broccoli will fight and/or help prevent anemia.

12. Maintain a healthy pregnancy
Broccoli is a good source of folate. Folate can help prevent neurological defects such as spina bifida in the fetus. All women need a viable source of folate during pregnancy.

13. Reduce Alzheimer's disease risk

14. Lower cholesterol and high blood pressure

15. Reduce Stroke and heart disease risk
Lutein is a carotenoid found in broccoli. It can help prevent the thickening of the arteries in the heart.

16. Weight loss diet
Approximately 146 gram of broccoli has less than 50 calories. Broccoli is a great choice for someone trying to lose weight. Broccoli is extremely low in calorie content.

17. Nervous System
Broccoli contains adequate amounts of potassium which helps maintain a *healthy nervous system* and optimal brain function which help promote regular muscle growth.

18. Blood Pressure
Along with a high amount of potassium, Broccoli also contains magnesium and calcium which help regulate blood pressure.

Caution: Phosvitin can stop iron intake by 28%. It is found in egg yolk. Heme and non-heme iron are reduced by **calcium**. **Phytates** (lentils, beans, rice) can reduce iron by 50%. **Polyphenols** like cocoa (90%), coffee (60%) and **Oxalates** can halt our iron absorption too. Ingest iron 2hrs prior or 2hrs after.

CANTALOUPE

I like cantaloupe. Sometimes I will eat it with salt and other times I will eat it alone. It makes me feel hydrated and energized. Cantaloupe has a number of health benefits. Some of them are listed ahead.

A. Excellent source of Vitamin A. Vitamin A is a powerful antioxidant and it is essential for healthy vision. It is also required for maintaining healthy mucus membranes and skin. Vitamin A can help protect from lung and oral cavity cancers.

B. This fruit is rich in antioxidant flavonoids such as beta-carotene and it can offer protection against colon, prostate, breast, lung and pancreatic cancer.

C. Cantaloupe has moderate amounts of potassium. Potassium is an important component of cell and body fluids and helps control heart rate and blood pressure. Potassium can offer us protection against stroke and coronary heart disease.

D. Cantaloupe also contains moderate levels of the B-complex vitamins, pantothenic acid, vitamin C, and minerals like manganese.

CARROTS

Benefits carrots can provide you with are ahead.

1. Improved vision

2. Help prevent stroke

3. A powerful antiseptic

4. Help prevent heart disease

5. Healthy appearance of skin

6. Provides vitamin B13 and vitamin K.

7. Help lower risk of breast, lung and colon cancer.

8. Anti-Aging. Helps slow down the aging of cells due to large amounts of beta-carotene.

9. Carrots can help prevent certain infections. They can be used on cuts; either shredded raw or boiled and mashed.

10. Cleanse the body due to the vitamin A assisting the liver in flushing out the toxins from our body. It reduces the bile and the fat in the liver. The fiber that's found in carrots can help clean the colon and hasten waste movement.

11.Healthy teeth and gums. While chewing carrots, they scrape off plaque and food particles from your teeth kinda like toothpaste on a toothbrush. Carrots stimulate gums and it helps produce a lot of saliva. Carrots are alkaline and that helps balance out the acid-forming, cavity-forming bacteria. Minerals in carrots help prevent tooth damage.

CHEESE: **#1 source** of calcium in the diet **by a mile.** Cheese helps lycopene & fat vitamins absorb. **Page**102

CHICKEN (5th highest **carnitine** source)

CHICKEN (5th highest **carnitine** source)

After I was diagnosed with MS, chicken, fish and steaks were the main meats I ate on a regular basis. Chicken is filled with the clean quality proteins I seek. I try to avoid buying frozen chicken from the supermarket due to the preservatives added to it. I prefer fresh chicken. Although I enjoy eating fried chicken, I know the health benefits of it are not the best. That is why I prefer broiled, grilled or baked chicken. Broiled, grilled or baked chicken can be prepared multiple ways. The cooking preparations I use are beneficial, healthy, simple and the crucial chicken *collagen* has amino acids. Health benefits you can obtain from eating chicken are ahead. I recommend adding grilled chicken to the #1 salad option found on pg 38. I use 35g of chicken breast.

1. Chicken can help build muscles due to it having a lot of quality protein and a small amount of fat.
2. It can keep our blood vessels healthy and energy levels high. It's a major part of *"The Clevon Diet"*.
3. Niacin in chicken can help guard against certain cancers and other forms of genetic (DNA) damage. Chicken is 589 per mg/kg in **sphingolipids**. Pg 208
4. Natural Anti-depressant that can increase the serotonin levels in your brain, enhance your mood, help fight stress and improve your sleep.
5. Chicken has a lot of trace minerals that give a *boost to the immune system*. The essential mineral phosphorus supports your teeth and bones, kidney, liver and *central nervous system function*. Grilled, broiled, baked or in a crock pot is what I prefer.

6. Chicken has amino acids that help child growth and development and has the *amino acid tyrosine*.
7. Due to the selenium content, chicken can cut the risk of arthritis. Chicken can help support thyroid, hormone, metabolism and *immune system purpose*.
8. Chicken can assist in healthy eyesight due to it's high content of retinol, lycopene, alpha and beta-carotene. *Chicken is rich in phenylalanine*. Pg 212
9. Chicken can cut the risk of heart attacks because it is rich in vitamin B1 and B3. Homocysteine is an amino acid that can cause cardiovascular disease if levels are high in your body. Eating chicken breast can suppress and control homocysteine levels.
10. Chicken contains magnesium and that can help females cope with premenstrual stress.
11. Chicken has the mineral zinc. Zinc can increase and help maintain a healthy appetite.
12. Eating chicken can increase testosterone levels and speed wound healing due to the zinc content.
13. Relieves stress due to pantothenic acid (B5).
14. White chicken meat is a better source of niacin (B3) and magnesium. Dark meat has more thiamin (B1), iron and zinc. B1 helps build *myelin sheath*.
15. Chicken broth, chicken noodle soup, chicken in a healthy salad or chicken with our meals; chicken often play a major role in our health and healing.
CLAMS (Clams have more iron and B12 than liver.)
   Know & choose the correct **natural irons.** Heme iron (found in animal foods) is absorbed by the body easier than non-heme iron (found in plant foods). I believe the high iron (132% = 23.8mg per 3oz), B12 (1,500%), selenium and zinc found in clams helped improve my health after consuming clam chowder 2-3 times a week after my MS diagnosis in 97. (*See Iron pg 150*)

EGGS (Sphingolipids need fat for proper absorption.)

After I graduated from high school, eggs were somewhat omitted from my daily diet. I had began the TV dinner, fast food and microwave your meal life. After being diagnosed with MS, I added eggs back to my diet regime. Boiled, scrambled or over well is how I cooked them. Scrambled eggs require the use of butter or oil during preparation but they assist in the MS fight too. Eggs are very nutritious. Eating eggs with black pepper, salt and butter has aided my *MS success. Salt is vital to success.* Eggs have plenty of fat-soluble **sphingolipids (pg 208).** However, the yolk has phosvitin. Phosvitin inhibits iron absorption. One boiled egg can reduce iron absorption by 28%. Do not eat eggs 2 hrs prior or 2 hrs after a planned iron rich meal. Iron is essential and it needs to be absorbed. See page 150

Eggs contain the vitamins A, B1, B2, B3 (niacin), B5 (pantothenic acid), B6, B12, D, E, biotin, folate and choline. The minerals found in an egg are zinc, calcium, iron, iodine, phosphorus, magnesium and selenium. One egg has all of the nutrients required to change a single cell into a baby chicken. Eating boiled eggs provide more protein than eating them raw. Cooked egg protein is digested casier by the body than raw egg protein but nutritional content is about the same. Benefits of eggs are listed ahead.

1. Healthy fats (*See Dietary Fats in Notes on pg 141*)

2. Eggs are the only non-fish protein with plenty of naturally occurring vitamin D. (**Phosvitin inhibits iron, calcium and magnesium absorption.**)

3. Eggs contain quality protein. All of the essential amino acids in an egg are in the correct ratio.

4. Promotes healthy hair and nails due to the sulfur content and numerous vitamins and minerals.

5. Pick *pasture raised* over *pasteurized*. One has twice as much omega-3's, 3 times the vitamin D, 4 times the vitamin E and 7 times the beta-carotene.

6. Eggs do not raise your risk of heart disease, they raise HDL (the good) cholesterol. Eggs may reduce risk of stroke. Pasture raised have *rich orange yolk* but pasteurized eggs have *pale yellow yolk*.

7. Eggs are *great for eye health* because they have lutein and zeaxanthin. Eggs boost *immune system*.

8. Helps prevent birth defects due to the vitamins and minerals that are necessary for a healthy baby. Folate, choline and selenium are the top necessities that are needed from eggs during pregnancy.

9. Choline is used by our body to protect the liver, cell membrane structure and help maintain healthy neurotransmitter functioning. One egg yolk supply about 300 micrograms of choline. Research shows choline helps *enhance learning abilities, improves reflexes, memory functioning, regulates the brain, nervous system and our cardiovascular system.*

Note: Meat, fish, beans, legumes, peas, nuts, wheat germ and spinach have choline too but the choline in eggs is more readily available for our bodies. **If a raw egg floats in water, don't eat it. The air cells formed in it confirm that the egg is old or bad.**

FISH (Bible Food: Page 130, Cod is 4th in **carnitine**)

I began eating fish regularly once again after my MS diagnosis. Eating fish just three times a week can help boost your *immune system*, assist in blood clot formation, help hormone production, balance your cholesterol levels, help prevent heart disease, reduce joint/muscle pain, support healthy brain and nerve function as well as fight depression all while slowing down the aging process to help keep your body youthful. High quality protein and Omega-3 fatty acids are necessary in my diet. Many foods contain protein but different foods will carry them in very different amounts. Salmon, tuna, mackerel and many other fish contain high quality protein and beneficial omega-3 fatty acids. Fish are known to provide high amounts of vitamins and minerals such as vitamin A, D, calcium and magnesium. In my school era, I ate a lot of bream fish. I had great memory and I was a fast track runner. (Smaller and young fish are healthiest. See) Fish can help...

1. Improve eye health
2. Reduce high blood pressure
3. Reduce the risk of leukemia
4. Reduce anxiety and depression
5. Reduce asthma & ADHD in children
6. Protect your body against free radicals
7. Protect digestive tract & fight certain cancers
8. Battle mental disorders & maintain brain health
9. Protect against high fat in liver & kidney cancer
10. Supports healthy skin & naturally slows aging
11. Fights *inflammation* and *auto-immune* diseases
12. Improve heart health & help fight heart disease

13. EPA (the appetite suppressing hormone leptin) can assist in weight loss/see **Menhaden fish** pg 51.
14. **Fish collagen** is a chief collagen. It's anti-aging antibacterial, bone/wound healing and 97% protein.

Based on my studies, consuming wild fish vs farm raised fish may be similar to consuming organic vs non organic. Ahead you will find a list of a variety of fish, along with their **omega-3** fatty acid content from greatest to least. Their content is measured in grams per 3oz. (**Sardines** lead most fish in nutrients.)

1. Sardine 1.95 (Pacific,Wild caught) (#1 in **omega-3**)
2. Salmon 0.68-1.83 (Wild caught) (#1 in **vitamin D**)
3. Herring 1.71-1.81 (#2 in **vitamin D**)
4. Fresh tuna 0.24-1.28 (Most tuna is red or pink.)
5. Halibut 0.40-1.00
6. Canned tuna 0.26-0.73 (#1 or #2 in **iron, tyrosine**)
7. Pollock 0.46
8. Flounder 0.43
9. Mackerel fish 0.34 (#1 in nutrient **bulk + variety**)
10. Red snapper 0.27
11. Cod 0.13-0.24 (#1 **fish source** for **carnitine**.)
12. Catfish 0.15-0.20

Anytime you hear "Omega-3 fatty acids", salmon and tuna will probably join the conversation. Many people like them both and may wonder which one is more beneficial for their health. Both are loaded with solid nutrition. Let's take a look and compare both fish based upon 1oz so you can decide which fish may be best for you. (**Krill oil** is on page 56. It is **low** in DHA which is a top omega-3 fatty acid.)

Salmon: (I usually broil my salmon. Page 180)
6 times more vitamin D
Double the amount of B12
More omega-3 fatty acids (1,095 mg vs 240 mg oz)
Both have low mercury levels but salmon is lower

Tuna: (I prefer red tuna: Bluefin,Yellowfin/Ahi)
Less fat
More protein
More B6 (nourishes the brain)
More niacin (lowers cholesterol)
Double the amount of selenium (for reproduction)

Both are pretty much equal in their sodium (low), calorie and potassium count. Both fish also provide plenty of phosphorous. If you're consuming canned tuna and want to get the most Omega-3 fatty acids possible, choose water-packed over the oil-packed. The oil will mix with some of the tuna's natural fat and once you drain the oil-packed tuna, some of its Omega-3 fatty acids will be lost down the drain. Since oil and water don't mix, water-packed tuna won't release it's precious Omega-3s like the oil-packed tuna will. Tuna is a good source of B1, B3, B6, B12 and it has plenty of folic acid in it. Tuna carries large amounts of vitamin B, D, K, calcium, iodine, magnesium, iron, phosphorus, potassium as well as a ton of selenium. Yellowfin tuna has more B vitamins than average tuna. White tuna has more Omega-3 than plain tuna. Tuna can lower levels of artery damaging homocysteine and it can help stop atherosclerosis. Red tuna has myoglobin. Page 123

Vitamin K is a vitamin essential in *strengthening a healthier myelin sheath.* There is a chapter titled *Notes* located later in this publication (*pg 146*) that will tell you more about the importance of vitamin K. I mentioned it here because this section is about fish and fish contains vitamin K. I will share with you the top 5 fish that contain vitamin K as well as the amount each provide per 100g based on a study I read. There are other fish that provide vitamin K but they may be well below 5 mcg. I decided not to list them with the higher than 5 mcg fish below.

1. Light tuna canned in oil   44 mcg
2. Anchovy fish canned in oil   12.1 mcg
3. Frozen fish portions and sticks 10.7 mcg
4. Mackerel   7.8 mcg
5. Albacore/white tuna (more expensive) 6.9 mcg

Mackerel is another common omega-3 rich fish that you may hear a lot about. It's no surprise that it made the previous and upcoming list below. There are different types of Mackerel and they provide different amounts of nutrient value. Below I have only three types of Mackerel listed and the vitamin A, C, Calcium and Iron percent value of one fillet serving according to a stat chart I studied.

	A	C	Calcium	Iron
1. Atlantic Mackerel	4%	1%	1%	10%
2. King Mackerel	58%	10%	12%	39%
3. Jack/Pacific Mackerel	2%	8%	5%	14%

Note: King Mackerel is higher in mercury than the Atlantic or Jack/Pacific Mackerel fish. Be cautious when you choose your Mackerel preference.

GARLIC

Garlic is a strong tasting vegetable that is part of the onion family. It is normally white, grows in bulbs and has a strong pungent flavor. Garlic is very powerful and it is a natural antibiotic that will continue to help heal and cure illnesses throughout people's lives. The garlic cloves contain many vital nutrients we need like vitamins, amino acids and enzymes. Like onions, garlic is strongest when the cell membranes are broken through the process of chewing, chopping or by crushing. The garlic then produces a very powerful antibiotic and anti-fungal compound called allicin. Garlic also contain sulfur compounds from the amino acid allicin, which is most noted for producing garlic's powerful odor.

Allicin is one of the main components of garlic that gives it its health benefits, including the ability to help prevent certain cancers. Allicin is produced in garlic when the garlic enzyme allinase is cut or chewed. However, when or if the garlic is cooked, allinase is then inactivated and allicin can not be produced. Before consuming the garlic it is best to allow the cut or crushed garlic to be exposed to the air for at least **five to ten** minutes in order for the compounds to become fully activated. Then it can better benefit and improve your health. Eating 1 - 4 cloves a day should be a good amount to ensure that you have enough garlic in your system to absorb all of it's health boosting properties. Eating fresh parsley can help remove garlic breath. *Garlic can boost your reflexes and cognitive functioning.* Benefits of consuming garlic are ahead.

1. Garlic can help *lower cholesterol.*

2. Garlic can help *boost your immune system.*
3. It eliminates harmful bacteria without killing the healthy bacteria as chemical antibiotics do.
4. The hot taste caused by allicin is responsible for garlic being anti-fungal.
5. It thins the blood which can aid in preventing heart disease, the formation of blood clots, heart attacks and stroke.
6. Destroy free radicals & reduce overall oxidative stress thus preventing types of cancer.
7. Help prevent blood clots and destroy the plaque that aids in the development of Atherosclerosis.
8. Lowers blood pressure, can help *clean the colon*
9. Help joints and may help fight osteoarthritis.
10. Garlic can help prevent certain cancers (colon, stomach, breast, esophagus and pancreas)
11. Garlic + citrus fruit equals a *nitric oxide* boost.

For those who are trying to avoid the loud smell of garlic, try taking odorless garlic gel capsules or the pill form. The capsule or pill is nothing more than a high potency aged garlic extract. Keep in mind that no garlic supplement can match or take the place of freshly crushed natural garlic. Natural is healthier and better absorbed than synthetic.

Note: 1. I blend one clove, wait 5-10 min, add OJ, drain and drink on empty stomach. **2.** Fish cooked with raw garlic cloves lower cholesterol *easier* as a team (Pg 191). **3.** Raw garlic helped correct the MS foot drag I had that plague many MS patients.

LETTUCE (Beans/lentils are higher in folate. Pg 96)

I constantly express the importance of consuming live enzymes. When I am discussing live enzymes, I will certainly point in the direction of green leafy vegetables. Many people like to obtain their leafy green vegetables by consuming salads. Most of the salads we consume will normally contain Iceberg lettuce, Romaine lettuce and on occasion, a person prefers kale. If you are health oriented, you might want to learn the nutritional value of each lettuce. (*Dark leafy greens will help clean your colon.*)

Statistically speaking, Romaine lettuce has more nutritional value than Iceberg lettuce and it can last a lot longer in the refrigerator. Romaine has darker green leaves. *Darker green leaves usually provide greater nutrition.* Many people prefer Romaine or Iceberg over kale for their salads, maybe due to the taste or texture. Kale has more nutritional value than Iceberg or Romaine. The following 3 profiles will show how they all compare. The chart is a side by side comparison of Iceberg vs Romaine vs Kale.

Iceberg Lettuce: 100 grams

- 14 Calories
- 2% Protein
- 0.7 gram Fiber
- 2% Calcium
- 3% Potassium
- 0% Vitamin C
- 16 mcg Folate **(7.3%)**
- 30% Vitamin K

- 164 mcg Beta Carotene
- 152 mcg of Lutein + Zeaxanthin
- 10% Vitamin A
- 2% Vitamin B6
- 2% Iron
- 6% Manganese
- less than 1% Niacin
- 1% Copper

Romaine Lettuce: 100 gram (Romaine has lactucin)

*Lactucin and lactucopicrin are the vital compounds of lactucarium. They work on our *central nervous system.*

- 17 Calories
- 2% Protein
- 1 gram Fiber
- 3% Calcium
- 5% Potassium
- 2% Vitamin C
- 136 mcg Folate **(34%, #1 lettuce for folate)**
- 128% Vitamin K
- 1637 mcg Beta Carotene
- 1087 mcg of Lutein + Zeaxanthin.
- 174% Vitamin A
- 4% Vitamin B6
- 5% Iron
- 8% Manganese
- 2% Niacin
- 2% Copper

Kale: 100 grams

- 50 Calories
- 7% Protein
- 0.7 gram Fiber
- 14% Calcium
- 10% Potassium
- 12% Vitamin C
- 16 mcg Folate **(7.3%)**
- 1021% Vitamin K
- 164 mcg Beta Carotene
- 152 mcg of Lutein + Zeaxanthin
- 308% Vitamin A
- 14% Vitamin B6
- 9% Iron
- 39% Manganese
- 5% Niacin
- 14% Copper

Per 100 g of :	Iceberg	Romaine	Kale
Calories	14	17	50
Fat	0%	0%	1%
Calcium	2%	3%	14%
Vitamin A	10%	174%	308%
Vitamin B6	2%	4%	14%
Vitamin C	0%	2%	12%
Potassium	3%	5%	10%
Iron	2%	5%	9%
Manganese	6%	8%	39%
Niacin	less than 1%	2%	5%
Vitamin K	30%	128%	1021%
Copper	1%	2%	14%
Protein	2%	2%	7%

If you plan on consuming fresh vegetables, eating them within a few hours of them being picked will provide the most nutrients. Most people purchase their produce from a supermarket. Be aware that most nutrient value in vegetables is lost when they are not exposed to light. Without exposure to light, green vegetables lose a lot of their nutritional value pretty fast because photosynthesis can not occur.

Photosynthesis is the biological transformation of light energy into chemical energy. The solar energy needs to be converted into a usable form of energy which is what photosynthesis does. Photosynthesis is the process of producing and releasing oxygen into the air. It is a process performed by plants to produce their own food requiring direct sunlight, carbon dioxide and water. Photosynthesis happens in continuous light whether your vegetables are in the supermarket, in your house, still in the ground or even if they are wrapped in a plastic bag.

How long have your vegetables been kept in your refrigerator? When at the supermarket shopping in the produce section, be advised that the vegetables facing the light should have the most nutrients. The green, leafy vegetables stored on the shelf exposed to the light in the supermarkets have more vitamins than the packages underneath or behind them that were kept in the dark. *Another salad that boost my health consisted of romaine lettuce, green peppers, black olives, provolone cheese and Roma/patio or grape tomatoes. Dressings aid nutrient absorption.*

Gen 1:30..*I have given every green herb for meat: and it was so.*

Note: Spinach has more vitamin C, K, magnesium and iron than Romaine. Has more *myelin repairing* folate than kale (3x more). I pulverize my spinach, kale, etc with a healthy juice then I drink/ingest it. Leafy green vegetables help boost our *nitric oxide.*

MUSHROOMS

After being diagnosed with MS in 97, I began to subconsciously consume mushrooms on a frequent basis. I began adding them to my chili, spaghetti, pizza, hamburgers, steaks, soups, gumbo, chicken you name it. I had become fond of mushrooms. I was receiving many nutritional benefits but at that time, nutrition knowledge was foreign to me. Due to the health improvements I received in 97, quite naturally mushrooms became part of my personal studies. I discovered mushrooms have a plethora of health healing properties and they are healthier for you when they are grilled or microwaved. I believe mushrooms definitely played a major role in my recovery. Some of the benefits that mushrooms can provide are listed ahead.

Mushrooms Can Help:
1. Lose weight
2. Improve bone health
3. Reduce blood pressure
4. Lower cholesterol levels
5. *Strengthen immune system*
6. Protect diabetics from certain infections
7. Improve iron, calcium, phosphorous absorption
8. Prevent prostate and breast cancer (White button mushrooms are the most promising.)

Mushrooms contain protein, dietary fiber and many essential nutrients. The vitamins Pantothenic Acid, B1, B2(Riboflavin), B3, B6, niacin, vitamin D and the minerals phosphorus, potassium, copper, calcium, iron, selenium and zinc can be found in mushrooms. Mushroom types vary in nutrition.

Mushrooms contain natural insulin and enzymes that help break down the sugar or starch found in many foods that we consume. Mushroom's benefits help with proper functioning of the liver, pancreas and other endocrine glands. This can help promote the formation of insulin and its proper regulation throughout your body. The natural antibiotics that are found in mushrooms can help protect diabetics from infections (particularly in their limbs) and painful, potentially life threatening conditions that could continue for long periods of time.

a. The mushroom that most people consume in the United States is the white button mushroom.
b. White button: #1 anti-inflammatory mushroom
c. Shiitake mushroom: Used for centuries by the Chinese and Japanese to treat colds and flu. 4 to 5 ounces a day can fight tumors. Has the most Vit D.
d. One medium **portabella** mushroom render more potassium than a banana.
e. Boiled mushrooms provide more antioxidants to your body than fried mushrooms.
f. Leave picking mushrooms from the wild to the professionals. Most species of mushrooms are not edible, are highly poisonous and look very similar to their edible counterparts.
g. Mushrooms with Broccoli is a powerful combination.

OATMEAL (Steel Cut oats barely win the oats war.)

Oatmeal was one of the foods/grains I consumed frequently during my very first MS recovery. It has a very wide spectrum of beneficial ingredients and health properties. Rolled, steel cut and instant oats have virtually the same nutritional value.

1. The fiber and nutrients in oatmeal can enhance our *immune system* response to diseases and it can help reduce the risk of certain cancers.

2. Oatmeal helps lower cholesterol, reduce the risk of heart disease and protects against heart failure. (*** *I often microwave my oatmeal with milk.*)

3. Oatmeal may reduce the risk of type 2 diabetes because the soluble fiber it has helps control blood glucose levels. *One of the healthiest whole grains.*

4. Oatmeal helps reduce high blood pressure.

5. Oats contain more soluble fiber than rice, corn or whole wheat. *The fiber helps clean our colon.*

6. Contains a wide array of vitamins, minerals,iron protein, complex carbohydrates and antioxidants.

7. Aid *friendly bacteria growth* and *weight control.*

8. Can improve memory and boost energy levels

9. Oatmeal acts as a *nervous system* stabilizer.

10. Can help clean and nourish hair, skin and acne

11. Phytic acid **binds** minerals like iron and zinc in **raw** oatmeal but **cooking** oatmeal **frees** them. Best to cook it. I often blend **1** cup of raw oatmeal, mix with my protein or meal replacement then drink it.

OKRA (Aka Lady's Finger)

Okra is a very important vegetable. It has vitamins A, B, C, E, K as well as calcium, zinc, magnesium, potassium, iron and zinc. Okra has fiber, folate and it helps lower cholesterol, fights diabetes, asthma, colon cancer, ulcers and constipation. Okra can aid our *immune system*, pH, heart, hair, eyes and sex.

OLIVES

I will briefly discuss olives here due to the fact I have a section on olive oil in the *Liquids* section found later on in this publication. Olives and olive oil both share similar health benefits. If you ever wondered what the difference in the health benefits of green olives and black olives are, the nutrition make up is nearly identical. The sodium content is the biggest nutritional difference in the two. Green olives contain about twice the amount of sodium as the black olives. The olive's ripeness when picked and the processing methods affect the color of them. Benefits that olives can offer are ahead.

1. Cancer prevention

2. Healthy skin and hair

3. Cardiovascular health

4. Great source of vitamin E

5. *Anti-inflammatory* abilities

6. Aids in keeping a healthy digestive tract

7. *Immune system help* due to high iron content

8. Eye health (fights cataracts, glaucoma and other eye concerns)

ORANGES

We all know that orange juice can be nutritious and good for our health. Orange juice can provide your body with B6, vitamin C, folate, phosphorus, potassium and thiamine. Unfortunately, sugars and other ingredients are added to store bought juices. Consuming fresh oranges provide more fiber than drinking orange juice. Citrus fruit assist in tyrosine absorption (*folate pg 212*). Try eating your oranges with edible flesh left on the fruit. Health benefits oranges can provide you with are ahead.

1. Good vision
2. Lower cholesterol
3. Alkalizes the body
4. High blood pressure
5. Relieve constipation
6. Fights viral infections
7. Protects against aging
8. Prevent kidney stones and kidney disease
9. Prevent cancer such as breast, colon, liver, lung, skin and stomach cancer
10. Has simple sugars with glycemic index close to 40 (55 is low). Diabetics should eat in moderation.

PAPAYA (#2 enzyme fruit, pincapple is #1, page 177)

Papaya is remarkable. After eating it, my walking gait noticeably improved. I learned that papaya is a solid, ample source of antioxidants, phytonutrients, vitamins & minerals. Papaya has the protease type *papain* and *special digestive enzymes* that deliver a mind-blowing effect both internally and externally. Benefits that papaya can provide are listed ahead.

1. Protect your eyes

2. Relieve muscle pain

3. Lessen the possibility of becoming pregnant

4. *Lower inflammation* (It improved my MS walk.)

5. Relieve digestion problems (Tropical Fruit heals.)

6. Lower your risk of many diseases such as cancer

7. Protect our heart with A, C & E by reducing the oxidization of cholesterol in your arteries

8. Improves your skin due to carotenoids like beta-carotene, lycopene and vitamins like C and E

PEARS

Pears provide a good source of fiber, vitamin B2, C, E, copper, and potassium. They are an excellent source of pectin and pectin is a water soluble fiber. Over 3,000 pear varieties exist around the world. Benefits that pears can present are listed ahead....

1. Antioxidants such as vitamin C and copper help make pears *a strong immune system booster.*

2. Pears provide lots of boron. Researchers believe boron may help our body retain calcium. If this is accurate, pears may aid in osteoporosis prevention.

3. Since our body absorbs glucose, pears can help increase our energy levels when consumed.

4. Pears contain a lot of fiber. Fiber is essential for a healthy digestive system. Fiber helps keep foods moving smoothly through the colon and it can help reduce the chances of developing colon cancer.

5. Due to the *folic acid* content, pears help sustain a healthy pregnancy if included in healthy prenatal diets.

6. This is because pears are a low acid fruit and are unlikely to cause any digestion problems in babies. Pear allergies are relatively rare.

7. The pectin that is found in pears help make the pears effective in lowering cholesterol levels. Pears are higher in pectin than apples.

PEAS

1. Peas are "Heart Healthy"

2. Peas are cholesterol free, low in fat and sodium and they feed your muscles and brain. Peas have natural sugar that provide your brain with glucose without causing a spike in your blood sugar level.

3. Good for your eyes due to Lutein

4. Our body cannot make lutein so we must get it from food. Taking in an adequate amount of lutein may protect you from vision loss as you age.

5. The pea is a starchy vegetable and a good source of energy, fiber, protein and essential vitamins. Peas can benefit your *immune system,* they have vitamin A, B-vitamins and contain nearly half your RDA for vitamin K (especially when eaten raw).

6. Cooked peas will provide more minerals that support your blood, muscle and bone health, as well as your *nervous system* than raw peas. Peas are rich in so many minerals like iron, calcium, copper, zinc and manganese. Fresh pea pods are an excellent source of *folate.*

BEANS & LENTILS ARE HIGH IN FOLATE

As a child I was anemic and sadly I ate very little *iron* or *folate* rich foods prior to my MS diagnosis. I now eat beans & lentils often due to **high** *myelin repairing folate* and *iron*. Ahead, I list the *folate* % for a few beans and lentils measured by one cup. Beans & lentils have way more *folate* than salads.

Lentils 90% Black eyed peas 89% Mung beans 80%

Pinto beans 74% Chickpeas 71% (*Nutritional value of* **canned lentils** *do not shrink but* **canned vegetables** *do.* I eat my **beans** with cheese to manage my MS health.)

POTATOES

I consume more potatoes now because of my MS diagnosis. I found out that root vegetables can help assist MS patients. Not to mention, potatoes are a very healthy food. Unfortunately, many people eat them in other forms like unhealthy french fries and potato chips. The baked potato is suppose to be the healthy route but they are usually loaded down and topped with unhealthy fats such as butter and sour cream. This method of eating it, make it a potential risk contributor to a heart attack. Try staying away from the deep fryer and all that extra fat. Potatoes with good toppings are a low-calorie and high fiber food that offer very significant protection against cardiovascular disease and cancer. I like white and sweet potatoes but I was unsure as to which one was more beneficial for my health. I am pretty sure that someone else has asked themselves that same question. Both potatoes share many of the same benefits. Benefits of both potatoes are listed ahead.

White Potatoes

1. Potatoes are good sources of potassium, which helps lower and stabilize blood pressure.

2. The vitamin B-6 present in potatoes is useful to protect against heart disease. Many flavonoids can help reduce the risk of cardiovascular disease by lowering levels of the bad LDL-cholesterol and keeping the arteries free of fat.

3. The high level of carbohydrates in potatoes may help in maintaining good levels of glucose in the blood. This is necessary for proper brain function. A slight increase in glucose could help enhance a person's learning and memory.

4. Potatoes contain carbohydrates which are easy to digest and they make digestion easier. Potatoes also contain a significant amount of fiber that aids in proper digestion.

5. Potatoes rich fiber content helps protect against colon cancer and the quercetin found in potatoes have anti-cancer and anti-tumor properties.

6. Vitamin B, vitamin C and minerals such as zinc, potassium, magnesium and phosphorus are very beneficial for skin care.

7.Due to the vitamin B6, vitamin C and manganese content, potatoes are great source to relieve both *internal and external inflammation*.

8. Due to the calcium, iron, phosphorous, zinc and manganese content the building and maintaining of bone structure and strength can be increased.

9. Magnesium can help prevent kidney stones by inhibiting the accumulation and buildup of calcium in the kidney and other tissues.

10. B vitamins help support our adrenal function as well as calming and maintaining a healthy *nervous system.* (*see Adrenal Glands pg 64:very important*)

11. White and sweet potatoes both provide B13.

Sweet Potatoes

1. They are high in vitamin B6 which help prevent heart disorders.

2. They are a good source of vitamin C which help fight the cold & flu. Vitamin C plays an important role in bone and tooth formation, digestion, blood cell formation and helps accelerate wound healing. Vitamin C produces collagen which helps maintain the skin's youthful elasticity and it is essential to helping us cope with stress. It even appears to help protect our body against toxins that may be linked to cancer.

3. They contain Vitamin D which is critical for the *immune system.* Vitamin D plays an important role in our energy levels, mood, helps to build healthy bones, nourishes the heart, *nerves,* skin, teeth and it supports the thyroid gland.

4. Sweet potatoes contain iron which aids us with adequate energy, improved red and white blood cell production and assists with resistance to stress, proper *immune functioning* and the metabolizing of protein.

5. Sweet potatoes are a good source of magnesium, the anti-stress mineral. Magnesium is also good for the heart, healthy arteries, bone and nerve function, blood, muscle, relaxation and is known as the *anti-stress mineral*.

6. They are a good source of potassium which help regulate heartbeat and *nerve signals*.

7. Sweet potatoes are naturally "sweet tasting" and have natural sugars that are slowly released into the bloodstream but without the blood sugar spikes a diabetic normally dreads.

8. Sweet potatoes are one of the best beta carotene sources. Beta carotene is a carotenoid and it is the precursor to vitamin A in your body. Carotenoids are powerful antioxidants that help strengthen our eyesight, *boost our immunity* to disease and they help ward off certain cancer types. They also help protect against the effects of UV rays and aging.

9. Helps lower the risk of rheumatoid arthritis and *chronic inflammation* of joints.

10. Sweet potatoes can help with stomach ulcers, acidity and constipation.

11. It has plenty of *folate* to aid in the development of a mother's foetus (baby in womb after 3 months).

PRUNES (Oxygen is crucial and it protects our eyes.)

I have always enjoyed prunes, raisins and most of the fruit in the fig family. I later became even more interested in prunes once I discovered that they are *oxygen rich*, contain plenty of vitamin K, can help fight heart disease and can help prevent type two diabetes. I drink ½ cup of prune juice on an empty stomach. Apple juice ½ hour later is fine. Prunes...

1. Help fight anemia
2. Help to lower cholesterol
3. Help prevent type 2 diabetes and obesity
4. Help prevent constipation and hemorrhoids
5. Help block cardiovascular heart disease, chronic diseases and cancer. Best to drink juice in morning.

6. Prunes and plums are high in soluble fiber. The soluble fiber helps keep blood sugar levels stable.

7. The soluble fiber helps you feel satisfied after a meal and can prevent overeating and weight gain.

8. Prunes and plums are the most effective fruit in preventing and reversing bone loss, hence reducing the risk of osteoporosis.
9. They are *loaded with oxygen* and a great source of vitamin K and beta carotene. *Nourishes my eyes.*
10. Prune juice is a rich source of anti-oxidants and aids in reducing signs of aging by making our skin look young. Best to drink it on an empty stomach.
11. Raisins have more boron than prunes. Boron is needed for balancing sex hormones, brain function, bone pain, teeth, metabolism of vital minerals etc.

Some people put prunes and raisins in the same category but they have their differences. Prunes are dried plums and raisins are dried grapes. Both are very nutritional. When it comes to measurements per cup, they are about equal in copper content but raisins have more calories. It's like 434 vs 418. Per 100 **grams** raisins have 100% boron, prunes 35%. Prunes take the lead in the other categories. Prunes have more fiber 12.4 vs 5.4 **gram**, more potassium 1,274 vs 1,086 **mill**, more vitamin K 103.5 vs 5.1 **micro** and more oxygen 5,770 vs 2,830 per 3.5oz.

TOMATOES (Spaghetti has been a blessing to me.)

Tomatoes are very nutritional and they can be very beneficial to your health. Did you know tomatoes are considered fruit now? The U.S. Supreme Court declared the tomato a vegetable in 1893 but things have changed since then. I still refer to tomatoes as vegetables. Health benefits tomatoes can provide and what they can fight are ahead.

1. **Anti-oxidant**:Tomatoes contain vitamins A and C. The cooking heat will destroy the vitamin C but vitamin A is pretty stable when heated.
2.**Diabetes**: Tomatoes can help fight diabetes due to the chromium content found in them.
3.**Cancer**: Lycopene content in tomatoes can help lessen the development of prostate, stomach and colorectal cancer. Cooking tomatoes will increase more of the antioxidant lycopene.
4. **Vision**: Tomatoes can improve vision because of the high vitamin A. A and C helps **collagen** absorb.

5. **Heart troubles**: Tomatoes can help lower blood pressure, lower high cholesterol and they can help prevent heart attacks and strokes because of their vitamin B and potassium content.

6. **Skin care**: Thanks to high amounts of lycopene, tomatoes are great for skin care.

7. **Hair**: Tomatoes can keep your hair shiny, strong and healthy plus help nourish your teeth, skin, eyes and bones. Lycopene is vital to my diet on pg 173.

8. **Bones:** Tomatoes can help strengthen and repair bone tissue/brittle bones due to their vitamin K and calcium totals. Parmesan, is #1 *cheese* for *calcium*. **1** scoop of Isopure has 30% *calcium*. (Page 40, 135)

9. **Kidney stones and gallstones**: Eating tomatoes without the seeds has been shown in some studies to lessen the risk of gallstones and kidney stones.

10. **Smoking**: Tomatoes can possibly help decrease the damage smoking can cause to the human body.

Lycopene (**top**:tomato juice, paste, ketchup, spaghetti)

Lycopene rich foods are normally rich in vitamin A, C, folate and potassium. Lycopene can also help lessen the chances of prostate, colorectal, stomach, skin, lung and even cervical cancer. The fat-soluble vitamins can stay in our system for weeks or even months. I put *cheese* and *parsley* in my *spaghetti*. I add meat for *selenium* and *tyrosine*. (Page 56, 212)

Lycopene is effective in maintaining the thickness and fluidity of our cell membrane. Cell membranes allow good nutrients in our cells and prevent toxins from entering our cells. A healthy cell membrane is needed to prevent multiple diseases and ailments. This *powerful antioxidant* can fight the following:

FOODS -TOMATOES

1. Infertility
2. Heart disease
3. Helps prevent diabetes
4. Helps prevent cataracts
5. Helps prevent the aging of skin
6. Helps protect your skin from sunburn
7. Lycopene can also help prevent osteoporosis
8. Helps prevent age-related macular degeneration
9. Lycopene is a *superhero antioxidant* detected in:

Tomatoes (Cooking them produce more lycopene.)

Pink Grapefruits, Guava, Watermelon, Papaya

Rosehip, Mango, Basil, Parsley, Asparagus, Carrot

Gac Fruit (Aka Jack Fruit) I buy it at Asian markets.
1. 10 **x** Beta Carotene *of carrots* **2.** 12 **x** Lycopene *of tomatoes* **3.** 40 **x** Vitamin C *of oranges* **4.** Has 40 **x** the Zeaxanthin *of corn* **5.** *Anti-aging* **6.** *Anti-inflammatory* **7.** *Antioxidant rich* **8.** *Destroys cancer cells* **9.** *Boosts immune system* **10.** *Fights bacteria and viruses* .
11. *Defends against cellular damage*

" *Lycopene is important but it is not essential.* "

Note: Lycopene **absorbs best** if eaten with a little fat/extra virgin olive oil. Lycopene is available as a dietary supplement but it doesn't provide the same nutrients or absorb as well as natural lycopene.

WATERMELON

Many people love watermelon. When consuming this great tasting fruit, you are receiving a number of healthy benefits along with that sweet taste.

1. Watermelon keeps your body hydrated.
2. The potassium that watermelon has can remove toxic elements from the body and it abandons renal calculi which is produced in the body and reduces the percentage of uric acid present in blood. When mineral contents of a watermelon and water began cleaning our kidneys, frequent urination occurs.
3. Watermelons are full of water but low in calories which mean they can help aid in reducing weight.
4. Contains a nice amount of Vitamin B6 which is helpful in increasing brain power. Brain chemicals are produced by eating watermelon which reduces stress and depression. Watermelon can help allow you to sleep more peaceful and sound.
5. Watermelon contains lycopene. UV rays damage your skin but lycopene gives protection against UV rays. Watermelon can raise *nitric oxide* production.
6. Due to the antioxidant and flavonoid content, it can offer protection against certain cancers such as colon, breast, lung and pancreatic cancer. It is also rich in *citrulline*, a *viagra like male libido* booster.
7. The content of Vitamin A in watermelon is good for eye sight. It *creates immunity* and also protects skin and mucus membranes.
8. Watermelon has adequate amounts of potassium which help in curing heart disease and keeping our heart healthy.

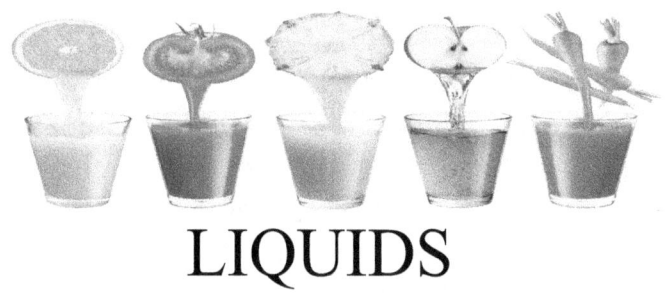

LIQUIDS

ACTIVATED CHARCOAL

When some people hear the word charcoal, they are not aware that all charcoal is not created equal. There is regular charcoal and there is the activated charcoal. Most people are familiar with the regular charcoal in reference to cooking BBQ. It can be used to remove odors, make art work and it has additional uses. While they both are derived from carbon, the activated charcoal type (also known as activated carbon) is a lot more porous than regular charcoal. Due to activated charcoal's larger surface area and the ability to filter out toxins and other harmful agents from our bodies, activated charcoal is the charcoal sought after for it's health purposes. Activated charcoal has oxygen added to it and is normally used to remove chemicals, toxins, and gases. If you need a colon cleanse, liver cleanse, kidney cleanse, a full body cleansing or a poison detox, activated charcoal is known to be the best detoxifier for a whole body cleansing. Activated charcoal assisted me with a improved walking gait and it helped neutralize the infamous MS foot drag that often plague many MS patients. I wonder if I had excessive amounts of aluminum in my body.

If you are guilty of unhealthy eating and you are trying to cleanse your body, activated charcoal can help assist in recovery. Water is the best cleansing agent to add to the activated charcoal. As it passes through the **GI** tract, it will be eliminating toxins and bacteria. While charcoal absorbs these toxins, your body will still need help to move the contents in your stomach along the digestive tract until all contents are eliminated from the body. This is why drinking plenty of water is very important.

Some people take activated charcoal daily and some take it two days a week. I sometimes take it twice a week myself. It depends on the individual. Some people will take it daily, cycle off after a few months then return after a one month break. I put one teaspoon of ACT in 8-10 oz cup of water then mix. Once I drink that, I add 8-10 oz extra water to the remaining activated charcoal in the cup. Be careful when opening your charcoal because it can easily "puff" and make a mess. Over the sink or kitchen table might be your best places to prepare your drink. Secure the top lid as soon as possible to avoid your charcoal trying to absorb odors and other substances in the air. The powder is reported to be more potent than the capsules and I agree. I got faster and better results from the powder. One advantage the capsules have over the powder is the capsules are easier to use, more convenient and not messy at all. Drinking activated charcoal can help lower **histamine**. Our bodies release higher levels of it naturally about **2 hrs** after meals and **at night**. **To much** can be harmful. I drink ACT at bedtime.

LIQUIDS - ACTIVATED CHARCOAL

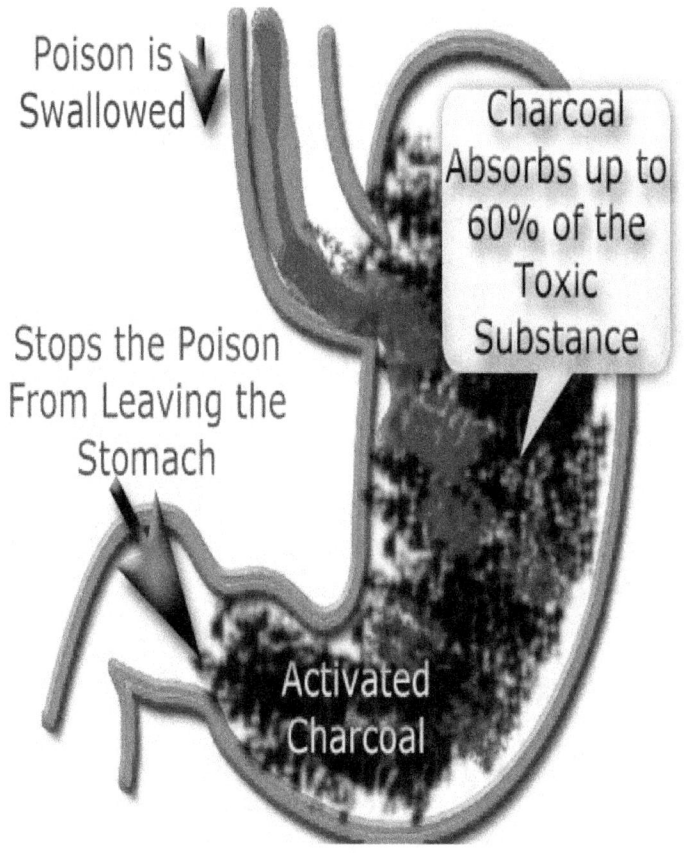

Poison is
Swallowed

Charcoal
Absorbs up to
60% of the
Toxic
Substance

Stops the Poison
From Leaving the
Stomach

Activated
Charcoal

Histamine-a chemical found throughout the body's cells and it works with nerves to initiate symptoms of allergens, itching, sneezing etc. Histamine is the *signaling chemical* our *immune system* releases.

Many medical professionals have used activated charcoal to treat drug overdose and poisoning in patients due to its ability to bind like a magnet to the toxins in the stomach in an effort to prevent the body from absorbing the toxins. There are so many uses and benefits that activated charcoal can offer.

What Activated Charcoal can fight, relieve or do.

1. Gout
2. Crohn's
3. Vomiting
4. Food poisoning
5. Dental infections
6. *Inflammation*, pain relief
7. Body odor and bad breath
8. Overall body detoxification
9. Various skin ailments, cellulitis
10. Hepatitis: chronic and acute viral
11. Poison ivy, insect bites, infected wounds
12. Relieve intoxication caused by chemotherapy or radiotherapy
13. Help lower cholesterol, triglycerides and lipids found in the blood.
14. Treating acid reflux or stomach pain caused by excess gas, diarrhea, or indigestion.
15. Helps rid body of poisoning by various drugs, alkaloids, chemical substances, toxic heavy metals.

Note: Many of the same materials used in making activated charcoal are also used to make the BBQ charcoal briquettes. Charcoal briquettes *are not* the same as activated charcoal and they *can be toxic* if ingested. Drinking charcoal might sound odd **but** at **7-8 yrs** old, I put ½ **tsp** of kerosene in 1 **tsp** of sugar. I **lit** a lighter under the spoon, I let it flame, cool then gel. I ate two. No side-effects. Decades later, I still haven't had a major virus. This was **created to kill viruses**. It's my personal supplement. I've ate 3 in my life. Pg 180
(For decades, my family has used kerosene heaters to heat our home. Kerosene heaters are kinda rare now.)

Apple Cider Vinegar With The Mother

Apple cider vinegar "with the mother" has a very strong taste to it but it has many health benefits. To gain these health benefits one needs to buy the raw non-distilled variety which comes with the mother. You may be asking "What is Apple Cider Vinegar with the Mother?" It is a non-distilled and organic natural cider. Raw organic apple cider vinegar is apple cider vinegar with the mother. This natural cider is rich brown in color. When held to the light, you should see a tiny cob web like formation of substances that as formed as it ages. This is what is called the mother. Natural ACV does not require refrigeration. You can save some of the mother and transfer it to other containers containing vinegar. Raw natural ACV has a pungent smell and can be a little to ripened. This can pucker your mouth and possibly cause some people's eyes to water. Do not let this alarm you because these are signs pointing to a good natural cider.

ACV is a strong detoxifier and it will help clean your insides. It can cleanse your body and kidneys while fighting chronic fatigue. It ranks as one of the premier natural remedies for healing the human body. Back when I had complications due to MS in 2014, Apple cider vinegar appeared to reset my walking gait once I consumed it. The results didn't last long but that was just a **1** tbsp dosage. I kept that in mind because I wanted a beneficial **daily** dosage. I believe apple cider vinegar helped expel excessive aluminum from my body. See pg 136 to better understand why I believe that.

If you are looking for great health benefits, avoid buying the distilled clear looking ciders. You can easily see those ciders do not contain "the mother". Natural apple cider vinegar that contain bacterial foam (aka the mother) have enzymes and minerals that you will not find in many other ciders sold in grocery stores. The mother is lost due to the over-processing, over-heating and filtration processes. The mother will settle down at the bottom of the bottle, so shake the bottle well before pouring. You *do not need to drink a lot each day.* I drink ACV 2 times a day. 1 tbsp with 1 cup of warm water in the morning, a cup at bedtime. The body feels full a lot longer, nutrient absorption is improved and ACV has the ability to protect liver cells. ACV can slow release of sugar into our bloodstream, helps avoid dangerous spikes in blood glucose, lowers body's need for insulin and it can take stress off of your pancreas. If our blood sugar is balanced we are less likely to crave carbohydrates. ACV increases your stomach acidity. This allows the body to produce more pepsin, the enzyme that will help break down protein. This action helps prevent gas and bloating. *Always drink ACV on an empty stomach or before you eat a meal.* For best results, *never drink ACV right after meal.* During detoxification, ACV will bind with the toxins which will help in removing toxins from the body. This can break up mucus in our bodies and *help clear our lymph nodes.* If you encounter bloating, have acid reflux, a stuffy nose, stomach gas, nausea or insomnia; drink 1 tbsp of ACV, warm water and honey before going to bed. *Natural ACV is superior to any synthetic pill form.* More Apple cider vinegar benefits are ahead.

LIQUIDS - APPLE CIDER VINEGAR

1. Fights allergies
2. Increases stamina
3. Helps relieve asthma
4. Helps relieve migraines
5. Can help reduce cellulite
6. Protect against food poisoning
7. *Strengthens the immune system*
8. Regulates pH balance in your body
9. Can be used for sore throat problems
10. Can ease arthritis, stiff joints and gout
11. Reduce sinus infections and inflammation
12. Fights warts and many fungal yeast infections
13. Used to treat skin conditions (acne, dandruff)
14. Effective as a body odor/bad breath remedy
15. Apple cider vinegar can curb sugar cravings
16. Can be used to balance high cholesterol levels
17. Improving metabolism to promote weight loss
18. Treat calluses, corns, plantar warts, fungus, etc
19. Some woman use in bath for vaginal infections
20. *Strengthens stomach acid* (HCL) to eliminate acid reflux and heartburn
21. Some apply to skin for a smoother complexion, sunburn, shingles, bites, foot and hand swelling.
22. Help dissolve kidney stones and helps prevent bladder stones and Urinary Tract Infections (UTI)
23. Kills yeast infections and fungus but it supplies the stomach with friendly, good bacteria and yeast.

Note: Apple cider vinegar, Activated charcoal and papaya have all helped my walking gait improve. I believe because they detox and fight inflammation. I blend my romaine, kale, etc (p 89 top) then drink my protein (p 157) 1**hr** afterwords for my gait too.

NEED HELP DETOXING?

If you are using apple cider with the mother as a detoxifier, I have some foods listed ahead to assist you in a detox. Detoxification is all about resting, cleansing and nourishing the body from the inside out by removing the toxins and then feeding your body with recuperative nutrients. A detox can help protect you from disease and renew your ability to maintain optimum health.

1. ALMONDS
2. APPLES
3. ARTICHOKES
4. ASPARAGUS
5. AVOCADOS
6. BASIL
7. BEETS
8. BLUEBERRIES
9. BRAZIL NUTS
10. BROCCOLI
11. BRUSSELL SPROUTS
12. CABBAGE
13. CILANTRO
14. CINNAMON
15. CRANBERRIES
16. DANDELIONS
17. FENNEL
18. FLAXSEEDS
19. GARLIC

21. GOJI BERRIES
22. GRAPEFRUIT
23. GREEN TEA
24. HEMP
25. KALE
26. LEMONGRASS
27. LEMONS
28. OLIVE OIL
29. ONIONS
30. PARSLEY
31. PINEAPPLES
32. SEAWEED
33. SESAME SEEDS
34. TURMERIC
35. WARM WATER
36. WATERCRESS
37. WHEATGRASS

20. GINGER;**peppermint and peanut butter can help get our sense of smell/taste back. Oils, wax melt too.**

BEEF/CHICKEN BONE BROTH & STOCK

As a child, if you caught a cold or became sick, chances are your parents fed you chicken broth or chicken noodle soup. Many people know that it is good for you but many don't really know why. As good as store bought broths/stocks are the benefits get better if you can make homemade broth/stock. The gelatin found in bone broth in particular is a hydrophilic colloid which is a watery, gelatinous, glue-like substance. Raw food consist primarily of hydrophilic colloids. The gelatin found in the bone broth is anti-inflammatory, it is nutrient dense and it contains a rich amount of minerals in an easy to absorb form. It also provides calcium, magnesium, phosphorus, silicon, sulfur and trace minerals.

My mother takes glucosamine and was amazed to find out that it contains broken down material from cartilage and tendons such as chondroitin sulphates and glucosamine. They are significant for arthritis, joint pain and they are instrumental for people who are suffering from *auto-immune, nervous system,* blood sugar, bile production and stomach lining issues. Homemade can be time consuming but it is fairly simple to make and so much healthier. When making your stock, the best part of the chicken are the carcass, legs and chicken feet. These parts will produce the most collagen for your broth. I learned that *chicken feet* produced the most. I purchase my chicken feet from an Asian market. The amount of filtered water should cover the bones. Add 2 tbsp of ACV with mother (best results), let it set for one hour, turn crock pot on high, then turn crock pot down to low once the liquid began bubbling. After

24 hours, your stock should be ready. The liquid needs to be drained and set in your refrigerator to cool down. A successful homemade stock will turn semi-solid in the refrigerator kinda like jello as the gelatin solidifies. If the stock does not gel, to much water was used or not enough collagen filled bones was used. Vitamin A, C, Zinc or whey protein help collagen absorb. **25-35%** of our body is collagen. Sardine is #1 **fish** in collagen but **beef stock**'s best.

1. It takes some time but it is super easy to make.

2. It is cheaper and healthier than store bought due to no excessive salt and added preservatives.

3. The calcium, magnesium & phosphorus in bone broth help our bones grow/repair. (**collagen**, pg 101)

4. The glucosamine in bone broth can stimulate the growth of new collagen, repair damaged joints and reduce pain and *inflammation.* Supports gut health.

5. Calms the mind and it can help you sleep better.

6. Fights allergies, cold, flu, eczema, leaky gut and it can help in the recovery from ***chemo*** or a ***stroke***.

7. Glutamic acid could be formed due to long cook times and agitate disorders **but** that is not proven.

Broth & Stock: (assists brain, heals gut, joints, skin)

1. Broth is made using predominantly the meat and muscle. (Chicken & Fish collagen are valuable. Pg 39)

2. Stock is made using predominantly the bones of the animal. It's **healthier**, more protein & less salt.

COCONUT OIL VS COCONUT MILK

I have tried to analyze the benefits of drinking coconut milk vs the benefits of coconut oil. I was trying to learn which would provide the best health benefits. Coconut oil appears to be more versatile than coconut milk due to the fact that you can use coconut oil in more ways than coconut milk such as stir-frying, sautéing, facial and skin care. You will gain more carbohydrates and protein nutrients from coconut milk. You will undoubtedly receive a larger amount of the health-boosting, much denser medium-chain fatty acid lauric acid from coconut oil concentrate. Coconut milk is *anti-inflammatory*.

Not many foods contain high amounts of lauric acid. Coconut oil is "almost half" lauric acid and it has about 6.5 grams per tablespoon. Lauric acid is a type of saturated fatty acid. A saturated fat can be detrimental in high quantities but lauric acid has microbial properties which means that it can help protect against bacterial infection. Lauric acid is considered the *"healthy"* saturated fat because it is a *medium-chain triglyceride*. Since lauric acid is a **MCT**, it is much easier absorbed by the body and has a host of many other associated health benefits. *Breast milk is the only other natural source that contains such high levels of lauric acid.* Coconut oil can be considered a *"superfood"* but limit your intake of MCTs. 4 to 6 tsp or 2 tbsp of coconut oil each day is advised. People who consume coconut oil often, get sick less. Choose organic, extra virgin or cold-pressed oil for best results. Benefits we can achieve from consuming coconut oil are ahead.

1. Reduce hunger

2. Can boost brain function in Alzheimer's patients.

3. Can help you lose dangerous, accumulated fat in your abdominal cavity.

4. Increase your energy expenditure which can aid in helping you burn more fat.

5. The fatty acids in the coconut oil are turned into ketones. Ketones can help reduce seizures.

6. Coconut oil can protect hair against damage, moisturize your skin and function as a sunscreen.

7. It can kill bacteria, viruses and fungi, helping to stave off infections like staphylococcus and yeast infections. Milk fights *joint pain* and *inflammation*.

8. Most saturated fats contribute to the cholesterol buildup in your body but coconut oil can improve blood cholesterol levels. It can help lower the risk of heart disease. The milk boosts *immune system*.

*NOTE: Some people are allergic to coconut milk but not coconut oil. Be careful if drinking canned coconut milk due to a possible BPA leach(pg 139). I did not mention **coconut water** in this chapter but it has more than 59 great health benefits. It is very hydrating, natural-not synthetic, it has electrolytes and was used for blood/plasma substitute in WWII.*

FULVIC ACID MINERAL COMPLEX

Fulvic mineral complex is a product that I have recommended many people to try for many years. I still remember the feeling of accomplishment I had years ago (2005) because I enticed a herb store in the state of AL to carry this product. It felt good to know that AL had one store location at the time to carry this product based upon the availability sheet and I was responsible for them carrying it. Fulvic is a very powerful detoxifier, helps one rest easier, heals wounds, stings, canker sores, anxiety, can be applied on the skin or taken orally. Over the years, many people have come to me and ask "Where can I purchase some of that Fulvic?" I discussed this product in *Your Health And Healing*. It was once described on my website as the miracle molecule on my homepage. Type the address below to enter the website for more information. This product has helped me, along with many others feel good and remain healthy. Fulvic Mineral Complex provides many helpful benefits. It can help heal so many different things, it has been viewed by some as a close "cure all". Ahead, you will find the fulvic mineral complex nutrition profile and some of the benefits this product offers. Vital Earth Minerals carry many outstanding products.

Official website is www.vitalearthminerals.com
1-866-291-4400
1-970-241-6628

100% Fulvic in solution - and nothing else!

Alkaline pH of between 7.0 and 7.8
Clear golden color; tasteless
Approx. 68 to 74 natural, organic
plant derived, ionic liquid minerals
from a fresh water source
Re-balance, detoxify, and energize
your body at the cellular level

Overview: Why Fulvic is such a powerful substance
Whole food, organic, plant based Fulvic minerals gently
extracted from rich organic Humic deposits. Minimally
processed without heat, pressure extrusion, or chemicals
of any kind.

The power of Fulvic Mineral Complex lies in the reactions it
enables within the body. Fulvic Mineral Complex does its
work inside the cells. Fulvic is nature's way of energizing
and balancing all systems of the body. It interacts with the
nutrients in food, and all substances within the body, both
good and bad; enhancing the good and eliminating the
bad.

Fulvic spreads through the system correcting imbalances,
restoring proper function of vital processes, and recharging
electrical potential of cells. As these corrections are
happening immune system function is elevated, and the
body metabolizes nutrients more effectively to facilitate
healing and rejuvenation of cells. Fulvic makes every
system of the body work better through its interactions and
reactions with other substances.

**Supportive research shows that consumption of
Fulvic:**

Enhances healing, repair, and rejuvenation of the
cells
Provides the most powerful anti-oxidant known and
is an incredible natural organic electrolyte
Heightens cell uptake- transporting up to 60x its
own weigh in nutrients into cells
Detoxifies the body of heavy metals and toxins
Increases energy and promotes sound restful sleep

Improves concentration, mental clarity, moods and
alertness
Boosts the immune system for protection against
colds and flu
Decreases body acidity to safeguard against
disease,
Helps convert sugars and starches to energy
instead of storing as fat
Decreases food cravings
Repairs and detoxifies the thyroid
And much more!

Fulvic: A natural, organic electrolyte
Fulvic is nature's way of re-balancing and energizing the
body. Fulvic bonds to and strengthens all biological
properties it comes in contact with. Fulvic can change,
alter, or combine with both organic and inorganic matter to
correct and enhance the biological performance of cells.
What this means is that fulvic electrolytes are literally
capable of restoring life to damaged cells.

Progressive stress, illness, infections, bad diet, and loss of
sleep all contribute to diminished cell energy. Left
uncorrected cells eventually mutate or die causing gradual
failure of organs, lowered immune function, loss of energy,
and more.

Experiments have shown ruptured and disintegrated cells
that naturally reconstructed and were brought back to life
when fulvic electrolytes were reintroduced. This means
fulvic has the potential to rejuvenate not only cells, but
organs, and all the systems of the body.

How does it taste?
All natural, mild taste; no sweeteners or flavoring needed.
Naturally processed without heat, pressure extrusion, or
chemicals of any kind. Many customers are surprised that
Fulvic Mineral Complex has virtually no taste. This is
because we don't use vile tasting chemicals during our
extraction. When you eat fruit and vegetables (the same
minerals you're getting in Fulvic Mineral Complex) there is
no bitter, terrible taste .

Any mineral product that has a strong repugnant taste has undoubtedly been processed with chemicals and you are tasting this residue. We are opposed to consuming chemical residues and any process that would damage the fulvic and humic. We absolutely never use this type of harsh processing.

Fresh water, organic Humic source material (100% from plants)

Our Fulvic is gently extracted from a rich, organic fresh water Humic source located high in the mountains of New Mexico. It is isolated and untainted by modern pollution. Fulvic is a natural component within Humic minerals; all Humic substances contain approximately 3% to 7% Fulvic.

Gentle, all natural extraction process
Because of our proprietary natural extraction method, Fulvic Mineral Complex has alkaline pH, helping to reduce body acidity. Fulvic neutralizes acids in body fluids, increases the absorption of oxygen, balances the metabolism of carbohydrates, and escorts free-radicals from the body.

Weight loss

Although we don't advertise it as a weight loss product, a great side benefit is that many people report losing excess weight after starting to take Fulvic. Body weight balances naturally because fulvic helps correct chemical and hormonal fluctuations, assists the proper metabolism of food, and diminishes mineral deficiency cravings. When these changes occur, blood sugar levels are balanced, and food is used for energy instead of stored as fat. Hunger is decreased along with cravings for high calorie starches and sweets.

Ingredients:

Fulvic/Bio-Mass Minerals: 18.75 mg
100% Fulvic in solution: Contains over 70 naturally occurring plant derived minerals, trace elements, and amino acids in an unaltered ionic solution.

Fulvic/Bio-Mass Minerals:
Antimony, Barium, Beryllium, Bismuth, Boron, Bromine, Cadmium, Calcium, Carbon, Cerium, Cesium, Chloride, Chromium, Cobalt, Copper, Dysprosium, Erbium, Europium, Fluorine, Gadolinium,Gallium, Germanium, Gold, Hafnium, Holmium, Indium, Iodine, Iridium, Iron, Lanthanum, Lithium, Lutetium, Magnesium, Manganese, Molybdenum, Neodymium, Nickel, Niobium, Osmium, Palladium, Phosphorous, Platinum, Potassium, Praseodymium, Rhenium, Rhodium, Rubidium, Ruthenium, Samarium, Scandium, Selenium, Silicon, Silver, Sodium, Strontium, Sulfur, Tantalum, Tellurium, Terbium, Thulium, Thorium, Tin, Titanium, Tungsten, Vanadium, Ytterbium, Yttrium, Zinc, Zirconium.
Amino Acids: Alanine, Glutamic Acid, Glycine, Histidine, Isoleucine, Leucine, Methionine, Phenylalanine, Serinine, Threonine, Tryptophan, Valine.
Other Ingredients: Purified Reverse Osmosis De-Ionized Carbon Filtered Water

Directions:

Adults: 1 fluid ounce, 1-2 times daily, as needed. Take with food for best absorption. Drink undiluted or add to non-chlorinated water, juice, or other Vital-Earth products. (The bottle lid is 1 ounce).
If health challenge exists introduce at 1/4 dosage to allow the body to detoxify slowly. Build up slowly to full dosage. Refrigeration is not essential, but is beneficial to protect the naturally occurring enzymes and vitamins.

Safety Warnings:

Precautions: Use only as directed. If you are pregnant, nursing or have a serious medical condition, consult a health professional before use. Keep out of reach of children.

GREEN TEA – BLACK TEA (Pu'erh) is fermented

Tea is loaded with antioxidants and nutrients that have powerful effects on the body. Improved brain function, fat loss, a lower risk of cancer and many other incredible benefits are benefits of a great tea. Many bio-active compounds that are found in tea leaves are the reason that tea contains such a large amount of very important nutrients. Try choosing a higher quality brand if possible. Some of the lower quality brands contain higher levels of fluoride. If you choose a lower quality brand, the benefits still outweigh any risks. Some people drink 3-5 cups a day. Black tea gives more of a energy boost due to more caffeine. Green and black tea come from the same plant. Both aid 1-15 but green tea is alkaline.

1. *Esophageal Cancer*

2. *Brewed cold tea has same antioxidants as hot.*

3. *Brain function*: enhanced memory and clarity

4. Improve *physical performance,* keeps the blood vessels relaxed and it can increase *weight loss.*

5. *Cholesterol:* Green tea lowers bad cholesterol in the blood & improves the ratio of good cholesterol to bad cholesterol. Cold brew green tea is sweeter.

6. *Diabetes:* Green tea may lower your risk of type two diabetes. Green tea can help regulate glucose levels slowing the rise of blood sugar after eating.

7. *Heart Disease:* Green tea has antioxidants in it that have been proven to help protect against the formation of clots, which are the primary cause of heart attacks. (pH:Green tea 7-10, Black tea 4.9-5.5)

8. *Blood Pressure*

9. *Alzheimer's* and *Parkinson's*

10. *Anti-viral* and *Anti-bacterial*

11. Increases our *stomach acid* (HCL) production.

12. *Anti-Aging Skincare.* If applied topically, green tea can reduce sun damage.

13. *Tooth Decay:* Catechins are antioxidants found in tea that can destroy bacteria and viruses.

14. *Depression:* The amino acid theanine has been reported to help with depression and it is naturally found in tea leaves.

15. Contains flavinoids that prevent the oxidation of LDL cholesterol, *preventing plaque formation on artery walls. Tea stops stone formation/sticking.*

MYOGLOBIN (**Carnitine** is an amino acid. Pg 182)

Myoglobin is an iron and oxygen binding protein *found in the muscle tissue of most mammals.* The more myoglobin, the redder/darker the meat is.The red liquid that comes out of the meat is myoglobin, not blood. It stores oxygen inside muscle cells. All blood is drained during butchering. Dark meat has 3 times myoglobin than white but it has more fat in it. Dark chicken has more nutrients than white. Try choosing grass fed meat over grain fed if possible.

High Myoglobin Meats per Mg/g

1. Red Tuna 25 (pg 81) **5.** Pork Tenderloin 1-3
2. Filet Mignon 8-20   **6.** White Meat Chicken 0.5
3. Pork Shoulder 2-4   **7.** Cod Fish 0.1-0.3
4. Dark Meat Chicken 1-4   (See page 58, 180)

HONEY (Raw honey (**darker**) is a #1 choice.)

  Honey has been used for centuries for it's health benefits. 2 tbsp a day for women and 2-3 tbsp for men is fine. I refuse to use *honey syrup*. I use 100% raw honey because it has many benefits that *honey syrup* can't provide. I add honey to my teas, lemon juice etc to replace sugar. Honey is natural and it is beneficial. Benefits honey can provide are ahead.

1. Heal wounds and burns

2. Reduce cough and throat irritation

3. Anti-bacterial, anti-fungal, anti-allergy

4. Prevent certain cancers and heart disease

5. Reduce ulcers and it is a valuable carbohydrate

6. Honey can improve our *immune system* and the honeycomb is edible. It can boost liver function.

7. Contain microorganisms that can provide health benefits when consumed called *probiotics*.

8. May help improve recovery from your workouts or help fuel your performance in sports. (Page 25)

9. Honey is nectar collected by bees from a variety of flowers. *Glucose*, fructose, and sucrose are the main sugars. Raw honey is lower in fructose than refined sugar, contain trace minerals and it absorbs slower than refined sugar. This gives longer lasting energy and a lower risk of a spike in blood sugar.

10. Honey has been said to help improve eyesight, assist with diarrhea, asthma, impotence, premature ejaculation, sleep, urinary tract infections, memory and help assist with weight management.

11. Raw honey contains intricate amounts of many vitamins and minerals such as zinc, niacin, iron, potassium, magnesium, manganese, phosphorous, calcium, copper, riboflavin and plenty of *glucose*.

12. Honey's anti-bacterial qualities are anti-aging and they can benefit us with softer, beautiful skin.

In the Bible, honey was a symbol of good health for Samuel (*1 Sam 14: 24-27*) and it was a honored gift (*Genesis 43:11*). John the Baptist utilized wild honey for food to survive (*Mathew 3:1-4*).

Proverbs 24:13 *My son, eat thou honey, because* **it is** *good; and the Honeycomb,* **which is** *sweet to thy taste:* (Honey's best consumed on empty stomach.)

Note: I soaked my steaks overnight with honey + wine ("late 90s, Diet #1 status", page 211). I never heat honey now. I add **1** tsp to my cold brewed tea.

WARNING: The health benefits of honey and the natural enzymes can be destroyed if heated to high temperatures. If honey is heated above 108 degrees Fahrenheit, it can become toxic to the human body. It becomes a glue-like substance that is extremely hard to digest and pretty difficult for our intestinal tract to pass. (*****1** tsp at night or in morning is great.*****)

LEMONS

Drinking warm lemon water can aid the digestive system and makes the process of eliminating waste products from the body easier. It will help prevent constipation, diarrhea and is often used as a weight loss remedy. Lemons contain small traces of iron, vitamin A and it plays the role of a blood purifier.

1. Lemon is an excellent and rich source of vitamin C, an essential nutrient that *protects the body from immune system deficiencies.*

2. Lemons contain pectin fiber which is beneficial for colon health. It also serves as a pretty powerful antibacterial.

3. It balances/maintain the pH levels in the body.

4. Having warm lemon juice early in the morning helps flush out toxins.

5. Lemons aid digestion, encourage bile production

6. It is also a great source of citric acid, potassium, calcium, phosphorus and magnesium.

7. It helps prevent the growth and multiplication of pathogenic bacteria that cause infections and diseases. *Lemon juice with olive oil is powerful.*

8. It helps in reducing the pain and *inflammation* in joints and knees as it dissolves uric acid.

9. Lemons can help cure the common cold.

10. Aids in the production of digestive juices

11. The potassium content in lemons help nourish brain and nerve cells

12. It strengthens the liver by providing energy to the liver enzymes when they are too dilute/weak

13. It helps balance the calcium and oxygen levels in the liver In case of a heart burn, taking a glass of concentrated lemon juice can give relief

14. Immense benefit to the skin and it prevents the formation of wrinkles and acne

15. Helps maintain the health of the eyes and helps fight against eye problems

16. Helps replenish your body salts especially after a strenuous workout session

17. Drinking lemon water often, can *help prevent as well as help dissolve kidney and gall stones.*

It is important to note that drinking lemon juice can ruin your enamel if the juice comes directly in contact with your teeth often. Make sure you rinse your mouth thoroughly after drinking. I use a straw if drinking pure lemon juice. Many people dilute their lemon juice with warm water before drinking. Lemons are acidic until they enter your body, then they become highly alkalizing. Try squeezing fresh lemon juice in water and drink it throughout the day for a healthy alkalizing drink if you don't want to drink pure lemon juice. I drink 16**oz** of lemon water frequently using pure or distilled water.

*Note: At times I add **1 tsp** or **tbsp** of ACV with the mother to my lemon water to enhance it's benefits.*

LIME

Similar to lemons, limes are also citrus fruits that are often sour but can be very nutritional. Some of the health benefits that limes can help aid you with can be found ahead.

1. Antibiotics

2. Eye health

3. *Immunity booster*
4. *Cancer prevention*

5. *Anti-inflammatory*

6. High in antioxidants

7. Rheumatoid arthritis prevention

8. Improves digestion and can lower blood sugar
9. Limes can help prevent mouth, stomach, breast, skin, lung and other cancers.

10. Lime-water juice can work wonders for people having heart problems. Lime reduces heart disease.

11. Vitamin C can *boost the immune system.* It also supports heart health, wards off sickness, diseases and it can aid in fighting cataracts.

MY TOP ROOT VEGETABLES

My top root vegetables I juice or eat are sweet or white potatoes, carrots, beets, turnips & radish. In *My MS Success* on page 135, I mentioned that B13 is found in root vegetables. B13 is important to MS patients. I put carrots, potatoes, onions in pot roast.

OLIVE OIL

Olive oil is clearly one of the good oils and it is known as one of the healing fats. This oil is a good source of the popular omega-3 and omega-6 fatty acids. When there are adequate amounts of Omega 3 and 6 in the body or a living organism it is then transformed into an omega-9 fatty acid known as oleic acid. Omega-9 helps reduce cholesterol, risk of cancer, prevents atherosclerosis and *strengthens the immune system.*

The greatest exponent of monounsaturated fat is olive oil. No other naturally produced oil has as large an amount of monounsaturated fat. Olive oil preserves the taste, aroma, vitamins and properties of the olive fruit. Olive oil is the only vegetable oil that can be consumed as it is, freshly pressed from the fruit. It is well tolerated by the stomach, has a beneficial effect on ulcers, gastritis and has been reported to help lower the incidence of gallstone formation. Studies show that two tablespoons of olive oil a day can offer protection against heart disease and help control LDL ("bad") cholesterol levels while raising HDL (the "good" cholesterol) levels. Olive oil is one of the healthy oils that can aid and assist with the proper absorption of many vitamins and minerals. That is why I drizzle it or a healthy kind of dressing on many of my *fresh daily salads.* Olive oil is very healthy and it can improve your health in so many ways. Some of the benefits you can obtain from using olive oil are ahead.

1. Treat sunburn
2. Aid in digestion
3. Lower your blood pressure
4. Cure or reduce certain acne
5. Can help fight breast cancer
6. Help increase your life span

7. Reduce bad cholesterol levels
8. Olive oil is a powerful anti-irritant
9. Help fight off degenerative diseases
10. Can help fight colorectal/colon cancer
11. Clean and inhibit skin from aging prematurely
12. Improve memory and maybe fight Alzheimer's
13. Two tablespoons a day can lower risk of stroke and heart attack (*best taken on an empty stomach*).
14. Activates secretion of pancreatic hormones and bile more naturally than some prescribed drugs.
15. This oil has *anti-inflammatory* compounds with potency and a profile said to be comparable to that of Ibuprofen. (*Lemon juice improves this benefit.*)
16. Two tablespoons a day could replace your daily vitamin E supplement.
17. Two tablespoons each day can lower the risk of coronary heart disease (particularly in women).
18. Some people drink ½ cup of olive oil daily, ¼ cup daily is adequate. If you mix 1 tbsp with 1 tbsp lemon juice, take on *an empty stomach* am **or** pm.
Bible Health Food: extra virgin olive oil, sprouted grain bread, fish, fruit, vegetables, raw honey

There are multiple choices to choose from when buying olive oil. Years ago, an employee could not assist me in buying olive oil because they did not know the difference. I went home that day, studied and learned about the different varieties. It is best to purchase olive oil in dark glass because light is an enemy to olive oil and it's great health qualities. The different varieties I studied are below.

Extra virgin- considered the best, least processed, and consist of the oil from the first pressing of the olives. Extra virgin is higher quality and has higher anti-oxidant concentrations and anti-inflammatory compounds (specially vitamin E and phenols). The less the olive oil is handled the closer it'll be to it's natural state, making it the best quality olive oil.
Virgin- from the second pressing.
Pure - undergoes some minor processing, such as filtering and refining.
Extra light- undergoes considerable processing & only retains a very mild olive flavor.

Note: Many type phenols are believed to decrease cancer risk, have antioxidant effects and can rid your body of dangerous free radicals that can harm your health.

Deuteronomy 8:8 *A land of wheat, and barely, and vines, and fig trees, and pomegranates: a land of oil olive, and honey;*

OLIVE OIL VS COCONUT OIL

Are you having a difficult time deciding which oil to choose between Olive and Coconut oil? Both have great health beneficial values, both are great for cooking and they both share their own personal traits. I'll let you make your own choice. I looked and searched around for a reliable comparison of the two. Below is a comparison by the tablespoon. (Turmeric is great with olive or coconut oil. Page 2)

Extra Virgin Olive Oil vs **Extra Virgin Coconut Oil**

% of mono sat fat:	78% vs	6%
% of polyunsat fat:	8% vs	2%
Heart Health:	great vs	varies
Saturated fat:	1 gram vs	13 grams
Calories:	120 vs	130
Total fat:	14 grams vs	14 grams

Weight loss: Coconut oil has been reported to have better weight lose properties than olive oil.

CANOLA OIL

Canola oil is great for heart health, fights type 2 diabetes, high blood pressure, has more fatty acids than olive oil & no cholesterol. It's smoke point is 400 degrees F vs olive oil's 375. Canola is cheaper but olive oil is superior in terms of health benefits.

ORANGE JUICE

Oranges are one of the most delicious fruits that are equally popular with adults and children. Every fruit has its own nutritional properties and orange juice is no exception. The nutrients that are present in oranges can help your body fight against severe diseases such as cardiovascular problems, cancer and gastrointestinal disorders. Consuming orange juice with a high-carbohydrate, high-fat meal can prevent the occurrence of inflammation within the body and help prevent the development of insulin resistance and atherosclerosis. Drinking some fresh orange juice allow nutrients to be absorbed into the bloodstream without them having to go though the digestion process. Some of the benefits you can get by drinking orange juice are ahead.

1. Reduce risk of heart attacks
2, Prevent kidney stones and ulcers
3. Can help prevent certain cancers such as breast, skin, mouth, colon and lung cancer.
4. Can help *strengthen the immune system* as well as fight the common cold and the flu.
5. Help treat anemia due to the quantity of vitamin C it contains. The vitamin C *aids in the absorption of iron* into the blood stream.
6. Oranges contain *anti-inflammatory* agents called flavonoids. Flavonoids work remarkable for people with arthritis and cane ease their stiffness and pain.

7. Citrus fruit help *aid tyrosine absorption*. Pg 212

8. The antioxidant properties of orange juice can help make your skin look younger and slow down aging effects.

9. Magnesium, the *anti-stress mineral* found in OJ helps support healthy blood pressure levels. I drink OJ mixed with 1 cup of blended oatmeal at times.

RED WINE

Red wine has been fermented and it has plenty of health boosting benefits. Wine has been used in the human diet for many years. Benefits of consuming red wine (in moderation) can be found ahead.

1. Red wine can help boost *nitric oxide* production.

2. The melatonin found in red wine is a potent anti-oxidant, it has cancer preventative properties and it is anti-aging.

3. A compound in red wine called resveratrol has been shown to increase lifespan in animal studies.

4. Resveratrol has been shown to protect against Alzheimer's disease and dementia.

5. It can reduce the risk of heart and cardiovascular disease thanks to the resveratrol it contains and the other anti-oxidants found in it.

6. A glass of red wine per day can reduced the risk of lung cancer by 13%.

7. Four or more glasses of red wine per week has been shown to reduce men's overall risk of prostate cancer by 50% and the risk of the most aggressive forms of prostate cancer by 60%.

8. Lower the risk of breast cancer. Drinking more than 1 or 2 alcoholic drinks per day could increase the risk of breast cancer in women.

9. Red wine can fight colds and improve sleep.

10. *Can fight inflammation caused by disease*

11. Lower LDL cholesterol, Increase HCL. Pg 41

12. I used *"a little"* to marinate steaks. Pg 125, 212

Timothy 5:23

Drink no longer water, but use a little wine for thy stomach's sake and thine often infirmities.

ISOPURE ISOLATED WHEY (I drink it slowly.)
(Isopure's nutrients aid tyrosine absorption. Pg 212)
Isopure isolated whey protein is the powder shake I mentioned multiple times during this publication due to it's many vitamins, minerals and high pH. It *raises our glutathione* and *sulfur rich* foods aid it. I know my 3lb jug had 6% iron years ago. I recently saw 0% iron was listed. Maybe *ferrous sulfate* was used for iron and later removed. Iron in the form of *ferrous sulfate* can harm your vitamin E. If I take a supplement form, I'll use *ferrous fumerate, ferrous gluconate, ferrous citrate* or *ferrous peptonate*. See iron pg 150. I take iron with Isopure or OJ. I add Vit D at times. (My **zinc** pill = 455%. Oysters pg 171)

NOTES

ALUMINUM (A neurotoxic rich material)

Some reports show that high levels of aluminum in the blood may be linked to Alzheimer's disease, loss of balance, a loss of bodily control, dementia, memory issues, mental decline, reduction of bone strength due to calcium loss and depression. Many of these problems are common amid MS patients. Certain foods contain higher amounts of aluminum than others. I consumed the majority of the foods listed ahead regularly prior to my 97 MS diagnosis. That is why I recommend reading all the product's ingredients before buying and/or consuming them. The more foods we eat with aluminum in them, the more metal we are putting in our bodies. *Cooking using aluminum foil adds aluminum to the food.* A higher temp equal a higher risk. (Veggies are worst.)

Note: The food listed ahead was reported to carry aluminum in them. Foods with a * behind them are foods I was guilty of consuming in excess prior to my MS diagnosis in 97. The RDA of aluminum is 60 ml. A meal using foil spikes it about 400 ml.

NOTES - ALUMINUM

1. Cakes *
2. Waffles *
3. Pastries *
4. Muffins *
5. Cookies *
6. Pancakes *
7. Brownies *
8. Cupcakes *
9. Doughnuts *
10. Pizza crust *
11. Corn bread *
12. Carrot bread
13. Salted snacks *
14. Flour tortillas *
15. Banana bread
16. Baking mixes *
17. Coffee creamers
18. Pickles and relish
19. Microwave popcorn
20. Dipping batter for fried foods *
21. Many type artificial colors contain high levels of aluminum. *
22. Some but not all cheese used in frozen pizzas contain aluminum. *
23. Cocoa * I drink both, 100% unsweetened cocoa and cocoa processed with alkali. The antioxidants in quality hot cocoa is about twice as strong as red wine, it can lower LDL, improve blood flow, lower blood pressure, improve heart health, may improve your thinking and reduce diabetic risk. It provides B1, B3, copper, iron, potassium, zinc and caffeine. *Cocoa has oxalaates. Drink lemon water/tea often.* (**Cacao** is more beneficial and bitter than **Cocoa.** Page 153)

Eliminating aluminum from your diet may not appear to be working if you are drinking alcohol, taking prescription/over the counter drugs or if you are consuming toxic substances of any kind on a regular basis. That's basically because chronic drug use and/or any toxic substance exposure may cause side-effects similar to the symptoms of aluminum toxicity. Don't mix prescription drugs with over the counter, the toxicity in the brain can rise to harmful levels. Foods can help remove aluminum from our body. **Top Picks:** page 112 #13, #19, #23, #29, #32

When the brain becomes overloaded and strained, it can't function at it's best potential until the intake of toxic substances are significantly reduced. In severe cases it could be two years before you can see noticeable results. Once your brain is able to expel the toxins, it can finally cleanse itself. Be mindful that some health conditions may hinder the brain's ability to cleanse itself. When the brain becomes dehydrated, behavior change in a person is normal. Caffeine overdose or most anything can become toxic when taken excessively.

Mercury does not appear to be as new to the news scene as aluminum. As you may already know, to much mercury can be harmful to our health. If you are cautious of consuming mercury, I have three fish listed ahead that are well known to carry it.

King Mackerel
Shark
Swordfish

BPA (Please read, it's very important.)

My sister and I stood in the kitchen talking and preparing food one day. As I made preparations to heat some of the food in the microwave, I noticed her interest in what type container the food was in as well as what was going to cover the food. She then explained some information to me on BPA that I was totally unaware of. After watching and listening to a video online about BPA, I became even more interested. I decided to study and do some readings of my own. The information I came across was indeed worth paying attention to.

BPA stands for Bisphenol A. BPA is an industrial chemical that has been used to make certain plastics and resins since the 1960s. In 2008, the possible health risks of Bisphenol A (BPA) made headlines. BPA is a chemical that has been used to harden plastics for more than 40 years. It is found everywhere. It's in medical devices, compact discs, dental sealants, water bottles, the lining of canned foods and drinks, and many other products. More than 90% of us have BPA in our bodies right now. We get most of it by eating foods that have been in containers made with BPA. It's also possible to pick up BPA through the air, dust and water.

The U.S. Food and Drug Administration once said that BPA was safe but in 2010 the agency altered it's position. Your next question might be "How could BPA affect my body?" Well, BPA has been compared to "a synthetic estrogen" due to the BPA molecule resembling a near carbon copy of estrogen. Top reasons why BPA could be of serious concern are ahead.

1. Hormone levels.
2. Manhood destroyer
3. Erectile dysfunction
4. Helps form estrogen
5. Decreases testosterone
6. Reproductive abnormalities
7. Brain and behavior problems.
8. Cancer (maybe even testicular cancer)
9. Heart problems. Studies found that adults with the highest levels of BPA in their bodies have the highest incidence of heart problems.
10. Some conditions such as diabetes, obesity and ADHD could be linked to higher levels of BPA exposure.

These are possible BPA risks and they may sound frightening but keep in mind that nothing has been established. The federal government is funding new research into BPA risks. The Food and Drug Administration recommends people to start taking reasonable steps to reduce human exposure to BPA in the food supply.

Connecticut, Maryland, Minnesota, Washington, Wisconsin and Vermont are just a few states that have laws restricting or banning the sale of certain products containing BPA. Other cities like Chicago and Albany and a few counties in New York are likely to pass similar laws. I also read that BPA is banned in European Union and several other major Western Nations. Eliminating BPA from your life is presumably impossible but here are some tips on how you can decrease a lot of it.

NOTES - BPA

1. Find products that are BPA-free.
2. Look for "BPA-free" infant formula and bottles
3. Choose non-plastic containers for food such as glass, porcelain, or stainless steel.
4. Do not heat plastic that could contain BPA and since heat can cause BPA to leach out, never use plastic in your microwaves. For the same reason, never pour boiling water into a plastic bottle when making formula. Hand-wash plastic bottles, cups, and plates.
5. Throw out any plastic products such as bottles or sippy cups that are chipped or cracked.
6. Consume fewer canned foods, consume more fresh or frozen foods. Many canned foods may contain BPA in their linings.
7. Some plastics are marked with recycle codes. Try to avoid plastics with a 3 or 7 recycle code on the bottom.

DIETARY FATS

Eating way to little fat can actually lead to health problems. Many vitamins are fat-soluble and they require fat to be absorbed into the body in order for them to be properly utilized. Your body needs fats in small amounts each day for normal function, growth and maintenance of body tissue. Our body's use of dietary fat gives sufficient energy, keeps our cells functioning and our *immune system* working properly.(*monounsaturated/polyunsaturated/omega-3*)

Dietary fat, which comes from the food you eat, is crucial to the absorption of fat-soluble vitamins such as vitamins A, D, E and K. These vitamins are stored in our body for different amounts of time. Your body can store fat-soluble vitamins anywhere from a few days to six months. They are absorbed by your small intestine, stored in your fat cells and any excess in your liver. Your body will pull them from your liver reserves if needed. Due to the slow excretion rate from your body, be careful with your ingestion of excessive fat-soluble vitamins because they can become harmful if you consume to much. People who are eating properly will probably have a three month supply of vitamin D stored in their body. Vitamin K is created by the bacteria in your intestines. It seems that our bodies would have an ongoing supply of vitamin K in storage but without an adequate amount of fat in your diet, your body can not effectively absorb the fat-soluble vitamins that are essential for your health.

Avoid unhealthy fats such as saturated and trans fats. Some great sources of healthy plant fats are seeds, nuts, coconut and the heart healthy avocado. If you choosing oils, pick the best healthy oils like olive, coconut and flax seed oils. You only need a small amount for proper vitamin absorption. It is not difficult adding dietary fat to your diet. Again, a handful of some sunflower seeds, almonds, nuts or avocado with a meal can enhance the absorption of the fat-soluble vitamins you are seeking. Pg 28

Some vitamins like the B-complex vitamins and vitamin C are water-soluble and do not need fat to be absorbed. Since they dissolve in water in your body, they can't be stored. Water-soluble vitamins need to be consistently renewed and replenished more often because they remain in your body for a very limited time period. When your intake is more than your body needs for immediate use, the rest is excreted in urine. This means that your diet should consist of a continuous supply of the water-soluble vitamins so that your body can have them available if needed. This is not the case with vitamin C since it is water-soluble. Vitamin C can be stored in the adrenal gland for 3 to 4 months. It is dangerous to take large doses of certain vitamins so consult with your doctor or a healthcare provider for questions and recommendations.

FAT-SOLUBLE VITAMINS

The previous section explained the importance of fat-soluble vitamins and how they are required for our bodies to support a variety of tissue and organ functions. Our bodies store the fat-soluble vitamins primarily in the liver which mean they do not need to be replenished daily. Again, because of the slow excretion rate from your body, be careful with your consumption of the fat-soluble vitamins. Excessive amounts can become toxic. You only need small amounts and cooking heat does not destroy them. I remember the fat soluble vitamins by remembering the word DEAK. Instead of a LEAK in the ceiling, replace the L with a D. *Isopure has adequate RDA of each fat-soluble vitamin except D.* Consuming a nutritional shake plus a nutritious bar can also help provide the fat-soluble vitamins you need. The fat-soluble vitamins are ahead in alphabetical order.

Vitamin A

Vitamin A is also known as retinol. Vitamin A can help support your reproductive, digestive, urinary and your immune system. Vitamin A is essential to the health of your bones, skin and eyes.

Vitamin A rich foods include sweet potatoes, beef liver, tuna, carrots, spinach, pumpkin, *dark green leafy greens*(collards, kale, turnip greens) winter squash, sweet red peppers, dried apricots and dried peaches, prunes, cantaloupe, mackerel, oysters and tropical fruit (especially mango).

Vitamin D

Vitamin D is *an essential vitamin required by the body for the proper absorption of calcium, bone development, immune function, healthy teeth and the alleviation of inflammation.* Vitamin D is often referred to as a pro-hormone instead of a vitamin. This is because the body is capable of producing its own vitamin D through the action of sunlight on the skin and not always through the food we eat. It is estimated that sensible sun exposure on our bare skin for 5-10 minutes 2-3 times per week allows the body the ability to produce sufficient vitamin D. Your nerves and muscles require an adequate supply of vitamin D to function normally. Fish is naturally rich in vitamin D. A vitamin D deficiency can lead to a *weakened immune system*, increased cancer risk and poor hair growth. To much vitamin D can cause the body to absorb to much calcium which can lead to increased risk of heart disease and kidney stones. Vitamin D can help assist those fighting *multiple sclerosis, cancer, type II diabetes,* etc. At times I get extra vitamin D from sunlight.

Salmon, mackerel, trout, tuna, halibut, sardines, flounder, sole, herring, perch, mushrooms, caviar, sunlight, tofu, cod liver oil, dairy products and egg yolk are all great sources of vitamin D. It is clear that fish is a premier vitamin D rich food. Vitamin D fortified milk and cereals can also provide you with vitamin D. I often take a vitamin D softgel.

Vitamin E

Vitamin E has antioxidant properties, therefore it protects your body organs, tissues and cells from the damaging effects of harmful free radicals. This can assist in preventing several health problems pertaining to digestive, cardiovascular and cancers such as breast, colon and prostate. Vitamin E also guards our system's immunity ensuring a healthier liver and better kidney functioning. It can nourish your skin and hair, delay the aging process, reduce the chances of blood clotting in the body, work to improve the functioning of our muscle tissues and accelerate the healing process while stimulating the generation of new cells. Women may have an interest in vitamin E because it has several weight loss benefits, helps in combating menstrual cramps and aids in a complication-free pregnancy. Vitamin E is also effective in improving fertility in men and it may be beneficial in preventing mental disorders like Alzheimer's and Dementia.

Good sources of vitamin E: Almonds, sunflower seeds, *dark green leafy greens* (like spinach, turnip greens, mustard greens, kale), tomatoes hazelnuts, pine nuts, pumpkin seeds, beet greens, canola, safflower, avocado, broccoli, parsley, papaya, dried apricots, wheat and plant oils (coconut, olive, flax, cottonseed and sunflower oils).

Vitamin K (Vitamin K and K1 are different. Page 51)

The human body needs vitamin K to promote the process of blood clotting, protect our bone's health and stop plaque buildup in our artery walls. I was seeking vitamin K to help build a *healthier myelin sheath*. (See *Brain Function* below.) Vitamin K is a fat-soluble vitamin. Make sure you include enough fats in your diet for proper vitamin K absorption. I stated in *My Ms Success* that I cooked my steaks, chicken, fish and other foods using garlic salt and parsley. *During my late 90's MS recovery, I cooked with dried parsley (rich in vitamin k) almost daily.*

Anti-Inflammatory

Healthy vitamin K levels have been shown to *fight inflammation* within the body significantly.

Brain Function

Vitamin K is essential for proper brain and nervous functions. The outer wrapping around our nerves is the *myelin sheath*. It needs s*phingolipids* (a critical fat-soluble molecule, see pg 208) to form properly.

Blood Clotting

Nose bleeding, heavy menstrual bleeding, bruising easy, hemorrhaging and anemia are indications that a person is deficient in vitamin K.

Bone Health

Vitamin K ensure healthy bones and tissues. Found largely in the sources ahead, even *lycopene*. Pg 102

Calcification

Without a genuine supply of vitamin K, the body is at significant risk of atherosclerosis, cardiovascular disease and stroke.

Antioxidant

Vitamin K hasn't been shown to be an antioxidant in the same sense as vitamin C and E. The primary or basic forms of vitamin K have been exhibited to protect cells from oxidative stress.

High sources of vitamin K can be found in: one tbsp of dried basil 36mcg, one tbsp of dried sage 34.3mcg, oregano 33.6mcg, dried parsley 21.8mcg (*Two tablespoons of parsley contain approximately 150% of the daily recommended dietary intake of vitamin K. Dried parsley has more vitamin K than fresh*) Dark leafy greens (*spinach, turnip greens, mustard greens, collard greens, beet greens and Swiss chard*), broccoli, Brussels sprouts, Romaine lettuce, asparagus, cabbage, celery, kiwi, cilantro, okra, green beans, cauliflower, cucumbers, onions, tartar sauce, tomatoes, black pepper, bok choy

Medium sources of vitamin K can be found in: green peas, blueberries, grapes, carrots, squash, cloves, chili pepper. I eat **miso** for K1 etc. Pg 179

Herbs, fruit and vegetables were listed earlier but there are other foods that contain high amounts of vitamin K as well. Tofu is a great source of vitamin K. Vegans regularly consume tofu for their protein. Fermented cheese such as specific Swiss cheeses or Norwegian cheese are also great sources. When it comes to grains, you can find higher amounts of vitamin K in wheat bran, wheat germ and oats than you can in rice. Sea kelp, yogurt, meats and eggs are all good dietary sources of vitamin K. (If I add dried sage to my shakes it is because I can swallow it easier than dried basil, oregano or parsley.)

Note: In one study, I saw thyme listed as a pretty high source of vitamin K. Another study suggested it carried very little vitamin K. Mistakes happen so we have to be very careful on what we read. I saw one chart list dried basil with 2,143% vitamin K content and cooked Kale had 1,021% vitamin K content. The dried parsley, dill weed, cilantro and chives all had to take a backseat after I discovered dried basil had a lot more vitamin K. Occasionally, I'd drink basil, parsley or thyme tea in the morning with raw honey. Basil is called "*the king*" of herbs.

HYDROGENATED OILS (Critical information)

Many people know that hydrogenated oils are bad for your health and they think they are avoiding these oils by not eating fried foods or other more obvious items. Unfortunately, many of them do not understand that hydrogenated oils can be found in virtually every baked, fried and sometimes even in some frozen food products in the grocery store. In every grocery store there is an aisle that has all the snack crackers. This is the aisle that has vegetable crackers, wheat crackers and also different types of cookies. This entire aisle is well contaminated with hydrogenated oils. This aisle could easily be called the hydrogenated oil aisle.

There are almost no food products on this entire aisle that does not contain hydrogenated oils. You may have to go down the aisle to the unpopular section, often located near the kosher foods. There you may find some crackers called Wasa Crackers. They are made without hydrogenated oils and they are baked, not fried (at least in the U.S.). So again, practically everything else on the aisle may contain hydrogenated oils in the product. That means every snack, chip, cookie, cracker, pastry and just about every baked good (whether it is sweet or not) will have hydrogenated oil in the recipe.

The problem is, many Americans are consuming massive quantities of hydrogenated oils and many Americans do not know it. They are eating potato chips, nacho chips and many other kinds of snack foods located on the hydrogenated oil aisle. As a result, they are getting atherosclerosis or a build up of plaque in their arteries. Over time, of course this leads to widespread cardiovascular disease. More importantly, it can lead to strokes, heart attacks and the need for heart bypass surgery. Conditions like this can lead to a setback in regards to good health.

I try to avoid eating any food products made with hydrogenated oils. This is perhaps one of the most important things you can do to prevent the buildup of plaque in your arteries. What can you do? It is simple. Read the labels. It is difficult to be healthy in our modern society if you don't make a habit of reading the food labels of every food you purchase and consume. Personally, I rarely purchase a food unless I've read the label. It has to meet my criteria of not containing certain ingredients. People refer to these type ingredients as metabolic disruptors.

Always read the ingredient label. What you don't want are hydrogenated vegetable oils and partially hydrogenated vegetable oils. Even if you choose a soybean oil or safflower oil, the type of oil doesn't matter if hydrogenated or partially is mentioned in the oil, It can harm you long term. It can help raise your risk of cardiovascular disease and harm your nervous system. This can shorten your lifespan. If I see that type of oil in the ingredients, I will return that item to the shelf. Food manufacturers will no longer sell me food with hydrogenated oil so easily anymore. I know the potential harm it can cause.

Many people talk about the danger of consuming to much margarine and butter. Is hydrogenated oils one of the reasons why? If my mother is shopping for butter and other similar products, she carefully reads the labels to make sure hydrogenated oils are not included in the ingredients. Reading the labels is just a basic recommendation to avoid increasing the risk of plaque buildup in your arteries.

IRON (Chicken liver has more iron than beef liver.)

Iron is critical in producing hemoglobin, a protein that helps red blood cells deliver oxygen through our body. All iron is not the same. Iron in the form of *ferrous fumerate, ferrous citrate and ferrous peptonate* won't harm your vitamin E like *ferrous sulfate*. Without iron, **everything** begins to suffer.

(**Products list synthetic iron used. Also see clams pg 76**)

1. Low iron causes poor absorption of B complex vitamins like B12 and the *myelin repairing* folate. See "Caution" on page 73 and #14 on next page.

2. Some iron deficient women may be tempted to eat red dirt, clay, chalk or even paper.

3. If the inside of your lips, inside of your bottom eyelids or gums are less red than usual, low iron may be to blame. Low iron can cause hair loss too.

4. Feeling weak, anxious, irritable or unable to focus may be due to an iron deficiency.

5. Suffering from iron deficiency anemia for quite some time, could cause irregular heartbeats, heart murmurs, heart enlargement and even heart failure.

6. Insufficient oxygen to your brain can cause the brain's arteries to swell and result in headaches.

7. Sore, inflamed, odd smooth tongue; weight gain, low energy, low body temperature? Check iron.

8. A woman's period should consist of two to three tablespoons each month. Excessive blood loss can lead to iron deficiency. Iron **needs** zinc. Pg 172 #5.

9. Beef liver has plenty of iron, B2, B3, B12, folate acid, copper, potassium, selenium, zinc, CoQ10, EPA, DHA and the vitamins A, C, D, E and K2.

10. To much iron is harmful. Resort to the RDA.

11. Heme iron helps non-heme iron absorb better.

12. Oxalates block non-heme iron more than heme.

13. Dark leafy greens, whole grains, legumes and clams are all rich in iron. Vitamin C, beef, poultry, salmon and citric acid help boost absorption. I take my multivitamin or iron pills with orange juice so the Vitamin C can improve the iron absorption.

14. To best absorb iron, avoid certain foods 2hrs prior or 2hrs after consuming it; *Calcium rich foods, eggs, soy, coffee, cocoa, herbal teas, berries, apples, beets, zinc, nuts, wheat bran, foods high in oxalates, polyphenols and phytates each inhibit iron absorption.*

MAGNESIUM (required for **thiamin** to absorb)

Many have said minerals are more important than vitamins. Let's take a look at the anti-inflammatory mineral magnesium. I have had this mineral on my radar since the latter 90s. I even had it listed in *My MS Success* as one of my heavy hitters. Known as the "anti-stress" mineral by many and it is referred to by some as the "master" mineral. Magnesium is *arguably the most important mineral in the body.* This mineral is responsible for innumerable bodily processes and it is needed for every cell function from the gut to the brain. It helps regulate calcium, potassium and sodium. Magnesium is essential for *nerve function*, protein synthesis, cellular health and is a vital component of over 300 biochemical functions in the body. Magnesium is necessary for the proper transportation of calcium across the cell membranes. Calcium needs magnesium as well as silica, vitamin D and vitamin K for assistance in entering our bone matter. Excessive calcium intake has been tied to heart health issues by remaining in the blood for to long. The calcium can calcify into arterial plaque so please be careful.

Many illnesses are associated with a magnesium deficiency Absorbing enough magnesium could be the solution to many of them. There are hundreds of millions of people who are not absorbing their nutrients properly. Approximately 80% of the very same people may have low levels of magnesium. A *deficiency in magnesium could affect your central nervous system in a negative way* and that is never good news. Magnesium can easily be found in a number of foods but it's usually in small amounts. I will share natural magnesium food sources ahead, followed by supplements you can consume to help avoid a magnesium deficiency. Total has 15% RDA.

Magnesium Food Sources
1. Avocados (one medium avocado has 15%)
2. Bananas (one large banana has 9%)
3. Cacao (dark chocolate, more nutritious than cocoa, 1-2 **oz** or 1 square of dark chocolate bar daily is fine.)
4. Equate (creamy milk chocolate has 45%)
5. Fatty fish (salmon, tuna, mackerel, halibut)
6. Green leafy vegetables (½ cup spinach 19%, #2)
7. Legumes (black beans, lentils, soybeans, peas)
8. Nuts (almonds, cashews, Brazil nuts, peanuts)
9. Okra (It's slimy texture aids digestion and joints)
10. Seeds (1 cup pumpkin seeds has 42%, #1 source)
11. Squash (1 medium squash has 8%)
12. Tofu (1 cup has 12%)
13. Whey (Isopure zero carb has 50% magnesium)
14. Whole grains (whole wheat, brown rice, oats)

Magnesium Supplements
All forms of magnesium are not absorbed by our bodies equally. The multivitamins that I have been taking for years has only 50 mg in each pill. Even then, the magnesium used in it is oxide. This form of magnesium doesn't have a good absorption rate. When I take magnesium supplements, my plan is to take 200 mg of quality magnesium two times a day. I take it with a meal or get it in small amounts throughout the day. Some people take supplements *on an empty stomach* for better absorption. Taking to much can cause diarrhea, nausea or ab cramps.

Magnesium forms easiest to absorb

Magnesium citrate – the most popular supplement

Magnesium taurate – helps cardiovascular needs

Magnesium malate – a fantastic choice for people suffering from fatigue

Magnesium glycinate – easily absorbs and one of the most bioavailable forms

Magnesium chloride – impressive absorption rate, best form of magnesium to take for detoxing the cells and tissues

Magnesium carbonate – popular bioavailable form good choice for people suffering from indigestion and acid reflux

Magnesium forms most difficult to absorb

Magnesium oxide – this is the most common form of magnesium. It is sold in pharmacies, it is non-chelated and possesses a poor absorption rate

Magnesium sulfate – called Epsom salt, fantastic constipation aid, overdosing on it is easy, has been considered unsafe

Magnesium glutamate and aspartate – components of the artificial sweetener aspartame, it becomes neurotoxic when unbound to other amino acids.

NOTES - MAGNESIUM

Magnesium RDA

Age	Male	Female	Pregnant
14-18	410mg	360mg	400mg
19-30	400mg	310mg	350mg
31-50	420mg	320mg	360mg
51-older	420mg	320mg	

Signs of a possible magnesium deficiency are:

1. Anxiety
2. Calcium deficiency
3. Constipation
4. Difficulty swallowing
5. Dizziness
6. Fatigue
7. Fibromyalgia
8. High blood pressure
9. Hormone imbalance/PMS
10. Insomnia
11. Migraine headaches
12. Muscle cramps
13. Nausea
14. Osteoporosis
15. Poor memory
16. Poor heart health
17. Potassium deficiency
18. Respiratory issues
19. Restlessness
20. Type II diabetes
21. Weakness

Magnesium enemies: sugar, stress, alcohol, meds

NIACIN (B3)

Like all the B vitamins, niacin plays an important role in converting carbohydrates into glucose and metabolizing fats and proteins. Niacin *helps keep the nervous system working properly,* helps reduce blood pressure, help the body make sex-and stress-related hormones and plays a role in increasing the blood flow to certain areas. Niacin can improve circulation and cholesterol levels (HDL). This can successfully reduce the risk of stroke, heart attack and cardiovascular disease.

Consuming to many foods that are high in sugar can cause poor niacin levels in your body. While niacin can indeed help improve skin appearance, excessive amounts can damage your skin, lead to liver damage and digestive problems. Niacin rich foods are listed ahead.

Chicken breast, tuna, salmon, mackerel,turkey,lean beef, eggs,cheese,green peas, mushrooms, peanuts, avocados, legumes, potatoes, sunflower seeds

THIAMIN (B1) is a vital nutrient that has a lot to offer the human body. It can help promote energy production and digestion. It improves appetite and improves memory. It helps prevent cataracts, heart disease, Alzheimer's disease and it is an anti-aging vitamin. It stimulates production of red blood cells, has a positive impact on the *nervous system* and it helps develop *myelin sheath.* Top B1 foods: Pg 173

Brewers or Nutritional yeast, yellowfin tuna, trout, salmon, pork chop,beans(Navy), cereal, nuts, seeds

PROTEIN (**whey** isopure scoop:12% **calcium**,Pg 53)

I've known for years that protein is essential for the development of bigger and stronger muscles. Until recently, I never really knew how important protein was for the health and development of the human body. Many people appear unaware that all protein is not created equal and that their digestion rates will differ. The digestion rates don't just differ in the meats that we consume but they differ in the protein shakes we drink as well. Quality protein is important to the human body. If you were unaware of protein's importance, you may look at it totally different now. (I use Body Fortress whey protein too.)

Protein is known as the "building blocks" of our bodies for a good reason. Proteins are the complex combinations of the smaller chemical compounds called amino acids. *Amino acids contain oxygen, hydrogen, carbon and nitrogen.* (**Isopure** is **my** #1.)

1. Around 60% of the human body is water. Close to 40% of the human body's dry matter is protein. Protein is very important to our body. Drink plenty of water daily when taking protein supplements.

2. Proteins are responsible for cellular and muscle repair, oxygen transport, binding and transport of nutrients, fuel, hormones, DNA, movement, body structure, enzymes and protein increase **dopamine** which aid motivation, arousal, sexual pleasure etc.

3. Protein is essential for providing our endurance, muscle and bone strength, *immunity* and it can be found in every single cell, tissue, muscle and bone of the body. **Dopamine** aid physical/mental health.

4. Our body absorbs the proteins we consume and turns them into specialized protein molecules that play specific roles in our body.

5. If your body loses more than 14% of it's protein storage, severe health consequences could follow.

Similar to antibiotics, proteins help our body fight infections. We should ingest adequate amounts of protein daily. A protein deficiency can lead to....

1. Fatigue

2. A *weakened immune system*

3. Loss of muscle mass causing physical weakness

Many people turn to protein drinks, powders, etc because it is difficult to get the large amounts of protein they are seeking through natural foods in their diet. As we all know, the natural form is more nutritious and beneficial than the powder form. As I mentioned earlier, every protein powder is not created equal and all protein powders are not easily digested by the human body. Isopure is the protein I consume regularly because it has 0g sugar, many vitamins, minerals, 4.6g of L-Glutamine and 50g of quality whey protein isolate per serving. Isopure protein has iodine & is easily digested by the body.

NOTES - PROTEIN

Protein *stimulates HCL production* but drinking **a lot** of liquids with your meals dilute your stomach acid and can impair proper digestion of your food.

The health benefits you can achieve by consuming whey protein isolate are ahead.

1. Losing weight

2. Lower cholesterol

3. Helps control asthma

4. Anti-cancer properties

5. Reduce risk of cardiovascular disease and lower blood pressure. *Zinc turn amino acids into protein.*

Whey protein isolate is often more expensive than whey protein concentrate. Isolate is definitely the higher quality protein and it has a higher biological value. Whey protein isolate contains more protein, has less fat and it has less lactose per serving.

Whey protein isolate is the purest protein that is currently available. *Whey protein isolate has been reported to provide immune boosting properties. It may provide protection against the development of prostate cancer and it enhances probiotic growth.*

You may hear some bodybuilders say they can't notice any noticeable amounts of gains in regards to muscle mass when they compare whey protein concentrate to whey protein isolate. Me personally, I prefer *immune boosting properties* that are found in the whey protein isolate because they appear to be missing in the whey protein concentrate forms.

Do not exceed the daily intake of more than 1.7 grams per kilogram of body weight daily. Excess protein in the body can result in your body losing amino acids and could possibly harm your kidneys with increased nitrogen. Take supplements such as whey protein isolate or whey protein powder if you need it in your diet. Protein boosts **zinc** absorption.

UNREFINED HIMALAYAN SALT (84 minerals)

Sometimes salt is looked upon as the bad guy. We need salt because it is vital to our health but choose the right salt. Salt is not only critical to our life but it is one of the basic elements of which our body is made of. Without salt, we wouldn't be able to exist. Our human makeup can be compared to a walking, breathing, salty ocean. We have salt in our blood, our sweat and even in our tears. Our blood consists of salt-like water and has a specific combination of vital mineral elements. Every cell in our body is dependent on the presence of sodium. *It is water and salt that energizes and activates our bodies. Without water and salt the solid matter of our body would be absolutely useless.* (No **iodine** is added.)

A significant reduction of sodium can be just as harmful as consuming excess amounts of it. Over consuming can cause high blood pressure, strokes, osteoporosis, etc and very little can cause spasms, irregular heart rhythms and even increase the risk of heart attack in hypertensive patients. How much salt should you consume? According to my studies, the average American's salt intake is two to three teaspoons a day. The American Heart Association recommend limiting sodium to less than 2,000 mg.

Himalayan salt is easily digested. It does not go through any processing stage that alters the natural makeup of the salt. Himalayan is natural and a lot healthier than iodized salt which has been stripped down and left with only two minerals; sodium and chloride. Himalayan salt has 84. In the publication *My MS Success,* there is a chapter titled An Eagles Eye. In DIET #1, I used garlic salt almost daily to season my food. The garlic salt had added **iodine** and was consumed in moderation. During that time frame, *my MS symptoms had drastically improved.* **Salt** is a crystal-like substance, abundant in nature. **Sodium** is a mineral, one of the chemical elements found in salt. Salt and sodium "are not" the same thing. Again, Himalayan salt has 84 vital minerals, not iodized salt. Seaweed and cod fish have natural salt and natural **iodine**. Both are vital. Himalayan salt hydrates. Sea salt can dehydrate. Benefits you can gain from consuming natural salt are ahead.

Alkalize the body - with stable pH, help eliminate the risks of serious and life threatening diseases.

Asthma – *reduces inflammation* in the respiratory system. The production of phlegm is slowed down so you can breathe easier. Some say that sprinkling sea salt on the tongue after drinking a glass of water can be just as effective as using an inhaler.

Depression – effective in treating various types of depression, can help you feel good, relax and sleep better at night. Red **miso soup** boost my MS walk.

Diabetes – can help *reduce the need for insulin* by helping maintain proper sugar levels in the body.

Heart Health – Himalayan salt can help reduce high cholesterol levels, high blood pressure and help regulate irregular heart beat. This salt can help prevent atherosclerosis, heart attacks and strokes.

Muscle Spasms – Himalayan salt does not only contain small amounts of potassium but it also can help the body to absorb it better from other foods. That's why it is so effective in helping to prevent spasms, cramps and muscle pains.

Osteoporosis – By drinking plenty of water and consuming salt in moderation you can help prevent osteoporosis. **Miso soup** is salty but very healthy.

Promotes – Libido, healthy sleep patterns, kidney and gallbladder health. **Iodines** added to table salt.

Skin Conditions – Himalayan bath soaks can help relieve dry, itchy skin as well as serious conditions such as eczema and psoriasis. The bath naturally opens up your pores, improves circulation in the skin and hydrates the tissues so that your skin can heal. Also reduces the appearance of aging.

Stronger Immune System – Allows you to better fight off *autoimmune disorders,* the flu, cold virus, fever and allergies. **Iodine** helps *immune system.*

Weight Loss – Foods eaten are digested faster and this helps prevent buildup in the digestive tract. If left alone eventually it can lead to constipation and weight gain. **Iodine** helps prevent thyroid swelling.

Mathew 5:13 *Ye are the salt of the earth: but if the salt have lost his savor, wherewith shall it be salted? it is thenceforth good for nothing, but to be cast out, and to be trodden under foot of men.*

SILICA (Water soluble orthosilicic acid absorb best.)

At the very beginning of this chapter, I discussed aluminum and the possible side effects of ingesting way to much of it. During my studies I found that silica may help to counter the effects of excessive aluminum in the body. Silica (silicon dioxide) is a chemical compound that is an oxide of silicon with the chemical formula SiO_2. Silica is necessary, yet it is often known as the *"forgotten nutrient"*.

Without silica, *there can be no life*. All creatures, insects, plants and humans need silica for stronger bones, smooth skin, shiny hair, beautiful nails and structure to stand upright. Silica can also normalize circulation, regulate high blood pressure, assist in the prevention of kidney stones and can help heal urinary tract infections. Like most minerals that are inorganic; calcium, magnesium, iron and silica are difficult to absorb in our bodies. Minerals need to be predigested or chelated. In other words changed by plants into an organic flavonoid form so that it can be fully absorbed by the human body. Since silica is a trace mineral, *the body only needs a very small amount of it to remain healthy.*

Without silica, our hair would not reach it's full potential and beauty. We would have brittle nails, rough/itchy skin, no elasticity in our connective tissues, we would have brittle bones and possibly osteoporosis because the renewal of the bones and creation of cartilage depend heavily on vegetable silica as a nutrient in combination with calcium. *Our immune systems would suffer and we would age much sooner if we had a deficiency of silica.* A deficiency of silica in the human body could result in arthritis, atherosclerosis, wrinkles, Alzheimer's disease and I'm pretty sure there are other ailments that could be listed in this lineup.

I have read great reviews on silica supplements. I have also read reviews that were not very good. In one review, a few customers had purchased silica supplements and they were alarmed once they read a list of possible side effects. Some of the possible side effects of their silica products included heart disease, vitamin B-1 deficiency and kidney failure. *Take supplements as directed!! Excessive amounts of the supplement can harm you.* Silica is naturally found in so many foods, why would anyone need a silica supplement? It's the bio-availability of silica, the degree in which a substance can be assimilated and used by our bodies. Many people don't absorb enough silica each day. *Stomach acid is needed to absorb it.* Coffee/tea *create plenty of stomach acid.* Drink in moderation. Tea is easier on our gut. ACV *with the mother* is what is used to absorb silica if I use the red dirt method (one tbsp of apple cider vinegar, 8oz water, pinch of red dirt, page 194). On page 109, I stated how apple cider vinegar *with the mother* possibly improved the MS foot drag I was having on that day. I think ACV helped the silica in my body absorb (from the foods I was eating) and maybe expelled excess metals. I prefer the natural alternatives when consuming silica. If you desire, you can buy **liquid ionic silica** from various herbal health stores. Ionic ensures the customer the silica is easily absorbed. Natural food sources you can consume to provide your body with enough silica are listed ahead in alphabetical order.

NOTES - SILICA

1. Alfalfa, Asparagus
2. Banana (a top fruit, absorption rate is low, 2%)
3. Barley (malted barley and hops beer are richest)
4. Beer (one of the richest sources, richer than wine)
5. Beets (see #15)
6. Bell peppers
7. Bread (whole grain provide more than white bread)
8. Fulvic Mineral Complex (it is ionic, see page 117)
9. Green beans (a top vegetable), Garbanzo beans
10. Leafy green vegetables (vegetables top the fruit)
11. Mango, Millet
12. Oats
13. Parsley, Pears, Peas
14. Raisins (dried fruit) pg 100 (I add raisin to Total.)
15. Root vegetables (raw carrots, onions, potatoes, cucumbers, celery; found mostly in the skin/peeling)
16. Rice (brown rice has more than white rice)
17. Soybeans, Edamame (never eat raw or the pods)
18. Wheat, Whole grains, Bran

Other ways silica can benefit you;

1. Help rebuild cartilage
2. Helps normalize bowel movements
3. Guard against the effects of coronary disease
4. Has been said to help eliminate metals such as mercury aluminum
5. Help restore the mucus membrane in the sinuses and respiratory tract
6. Help keep your skin elastic. Early wrinkles may be a sign of low silica

7. Aid in the repair and maintenance of vital lung tissues while defending them from pollution.

8. Help bones remain flexible to avoid brittle bones and help broken bones heal faster

9. Help stop the pain of osteoporosis and restore the body's self repair process

10. Magnesium, Vitamin D and Vitamin K along with silica are all important pieces of the calcium puzzle in building healthy bones.

11. Has positive effects on the lymphatic system as it decreases swelling.

12. Horsetail is very high in silica. Be sure to never ingest raw horsetail because taking them raw could hurt your stomach lining. Try ingesting the powder or capsule forms of horsetail.

13. It is said that men usually have a higher silica count in their bodies than women. Possibly due to the fact that men drink more beer than women.

14. Do not eat silica gel packets found in products.

TOP ANTI-INFLAMMATORY FOODS

Kelp, Turmeric (studies say turmeric usage rival potent pain pills, minus side effects), Wild salmon, Shiitake Mushrooms (I consumed a lot of Shiitake mushrooms prior to the Diet #1 status), Green tea, Papaya (helped my gait), Blueberries, Extra Virgin Olive oil, Broccoli, Garlic, Sweet potatoes, Leafy greens, Fermented vegetables, Beets, Omega 3

*Inflammatory foods:*sugar, processed food, alcohol, fast foods, soda, sat/trans fat, *white*:bread/rice/flour

TESTOSTERONE (Avoid High Cortisol Levels)

I discussed testosterone in depth in *Your Health And Healing*. If you missed it, I will discuss it once again here. What is testosterone? Testosterone is a naturally occurring male hormone that is necessary for many vital processes in the male body. A man's testicles make the testosterone in men. A woman's ovaries make testosterone too but in much smaller amounts. Testosterone production starts to increase significantly during puberty and begins to drop and decline after the age of 30. Testosterone increases sex drive and it helps build muscle mass but there is a lot more to learn about this hormone than that. Testosterone also plays an important role in sperm production, red blood cell production and the way men store fat in their bodies. A man's testosterone level will affect his mood for sure. Lower levels or a decline in testosterone can cause the following.

1. Weight gain
2. Lack of sex drive
3. Increase chance of heart attack
4. Loss of muscle mass and strength
5. Mood swings, depression, irritability or a lack of focus. Do not eat **high phytate** foods **with** meals.
6. Difficulty achieving erection. *Testosterone alone does not cause erections. It stimulates receptors in the brain to produce nitric oxide, a molecule that helps trigger an erection.* (Nitric oxide foods pg 172)
7. A Low Semen Volume. The more testosterone a man has, the more semen he produces. Men with low T will notice a decrease in the volume of their sperm during ejaculation. **High Cortisol = Low T**

8. Hair Loss. Testosterone plays a huge role in hair production. Although balding is a natural part of aging for some men, men with low T levels could experience a loss of body and facial hair as well.

9. Fatigue and Lack of Energy. If you are tired all of the time despite getting plenty of sleep, or if you are finding it harder to get motivated to hit the gym or exercise, low testosterone could be the problem.

Avoid: *vegetable oil, seed oils, flaxseed, trans fats*

10. Decrease in Bone Mass. Men with low T can also experience bone loss (Osteoporosis) because testosterone aids in both the strengthening and the production of bone. Older men who have had low T for years are more susceptible to bone fractures.

Avoid: *flavored yogurt that have no probiotics*

Men whose natural testosterone production has dropped significantly can use artificial testosterone to treat low testosterone which is often called Low T. Low T is often diagnosed when testosterone levels fall below a normal range (300-1000 ng/dL). A blood test (serum testosterone level) is used to determine the level of circulating testosterone. However, testosterone replacement therapy (TRT) does come with both risks and benefits. Please talk to your healthcare physician. With that being said, let's focus more on trying to help keep testosterone levels at a healthy range...**naturally**. A person must eat healthy to keep their testosterone levels ideal.

To help keep testosterone levels in good standings of course one needs to eat healthy. A healthy diet with efficient amounts of vitamin A, B, E, omega 3s, zinc and monounsaturated fats is a great start. Olive oil, canola oil, nuts and peanut butter are great sources of monounsaturated fats. It has been reported that many healthy foods such as broccoli, cauliflower, cabbage, Brussels sprout, kale, collard greens, turnips and radishes each can help stop the formation of estrogen in men. Consuming a lot of alcohol lowers testosterone. **Phytic acid/phytate** is found in grains, nuts and plant seeds. Pg 91, 167 #5

I am pretty sure you figured that exercise was going to be mentioned somewhere in this equation so here it is. As you exercise, do so with intensity. Focus on what you are trying to accomplish. Train your legs harder than your upper body but work the entire body out equally. Some quality exercises to perform: squats, step ups, bench presses, weight pull ups, back rows, military presses, dead lifts and chin ups. It may prove to be more beneficial to use heavy weights because while it may sound strange, the goal is to place stress on the central nervous system. I am pretty sure there are other exercises to help raise testosterone but I only mentioned a few. Please be careful and do not overwork yourself.

Make sure you get plenty of sleep. Less than 7 or 8 hours is not good. The more you sleep the more testosterone can be produced. That is why a male will often wake up in the morning with an erection. A lack of sleep as well as stress can raise cortisol levels. Higher cortisol levels inhibit the production of testosterone and you definitely don't want that.

Another thing we should keep in mind is to enjoy the pleasant sun. The sun will not only supply you with some vitamin D but it can also help increase your hormone levels as well. Also be mindful to wear boxers or loose underwear. Do not wear tight pants or tight underwear and do not take long hot baths. Never overheat your testicles. Hot baths can interfere with your testosterone production. Foods or nutrients that can raise testosterone levels are....

Vitamin A
Sweet potatoes, carrots, dark leafy vegetables, kale, spinach, Romaine lettuce, squash, apricots, mango, tuna, cantaloupe, sweet red peppers (Consuming to much **synthetic** vitamin A is dangerous.)
Avocado: magnesium, potassium, B, E, K and zinc

Bananas and *Pineapple* both provide the enzyme bromelain. Bromelain can enhance a man's libido.

(B2) Riboflavin is essential for the manufacturing of testosterone. A few top B2 sources from greatest to least are cheese, almonds, lean steak, mackerel and hard boiled eggs. There are many food sources that carry B2, just in smaller amounts. Foods such as avocados, mushrooms, broccoli and green leafy vegetables contain small amounts of vitamin B2.

Beans ~ Pinto, kidney and black beans all contain protein and zinc. Chickpeas and lentils also contain protein and zinc.

Beef has more B12, iron and zinc than chicken and it has the *master antioxidant glutathione*. (Pg 135)

Brazil nuts are high in magnesium, which can help raise testosterone levels.

Cruciferous vegetables such as broccoli, cabbage and cauliflower, rid the body of excess estrogen, therefore increasing testosterone.

Vitamin D – Salmon has more vitamin D than your average food by far. Wild salmon has more vitamin A than farm raised salmon. Mackerel, tuna, eggs, flounder, mushrooms and Ricotta cheese each have vitamin D. An egg's yolk has sufficient vitamin D.

Eggs are rich in vitamin D and supply zinc. Zinc is essential for optimal testosterone levels.

Essential Fatty Acids - Salmon, tuna, mackerel

Garlic can boost testosterone when combined with a high protein diet for a month.

Oysters are rich in zinc. Zinc can increase muscle growth, physical endurance, sperm production and testosterone. Phytate foods impair zinc absorption.

Zinc is an essential mineral required by the body to sustain a *healthy immune system*, synthesize our proteins, aid sense of smell, trigger enzymes and is useful in creating DNA. **3oz** oysters = 445% zinc

1. Without zinc, our body can't make *testosterone*.

2. Zinc helps the cells in our body communicate by functioning as a neurotransmitter. (See pg 135, 160)

3. Lack of zinc can lead to poor growth, hair loss, eye and skin lesions, diarrhea, depressed *immunity,* no appetite, a drop in muscle mass and *impotence.*

4. Consuming to much zinc can lead to vomiting, nausea, diarrhea, headaches, a loss of appetite and abdominal cramps. Most foods on pg 56 have zinc.

5. Deficiency in zinc for a long period of time can obstruct the absorption of the minerals copper and iron. Iron and copper **need** zinc for best results.

6. Animal sources of zinc are superior to their plant source counterparts. The best zinc food sources are oysters, beef, lamb, chicken legs, beans and dairy.

Foods To Increase Nitric Oxide Production

1. Arugula/Kale/Spinach 2. Beets 3. Garlic 4. Meat 5. Broccoli 6. Red Wine 7. Pomegranates 8. Cacao 9. Watermelon 10. Citruses 11. Nuts(walnut)/Seeds

Foods To Increase Human Growth Hormone

1. Algae	7. Fava Beans	13. Raisins
2. Beets	8. Lemons	14. Chocolate
3. Blueberries	9. Milk	15. Water
4. Broccoli	10. Nuts	16. Watermelon
5. Coconut Oil	11. Parmesan	17. Whey protein
6. Eggs	12. Pineapples	18. Yogurt *Kefir

19. Grass fed beef 20. Gelatin desserts

THE CLEVON DIET

People have asked me on numerous occasions if I would share my diet with them. In 2013 I obtained a copyright for my diet known as "The CLEVON Diet". I consume adequate fat in my diet because it assists fat-soluble vitamin absorption. Avoid stress and excess sugars. Add calcium, enzyme rich/anti-inflammatory food, B vitamins, folate, magnesium, salt, iron, selenium, tyrosine, carnitine, zinc, D etc.

Clevon Harris "I consume oxygen rich food a lot."

Miracleintentions@yahoo.com

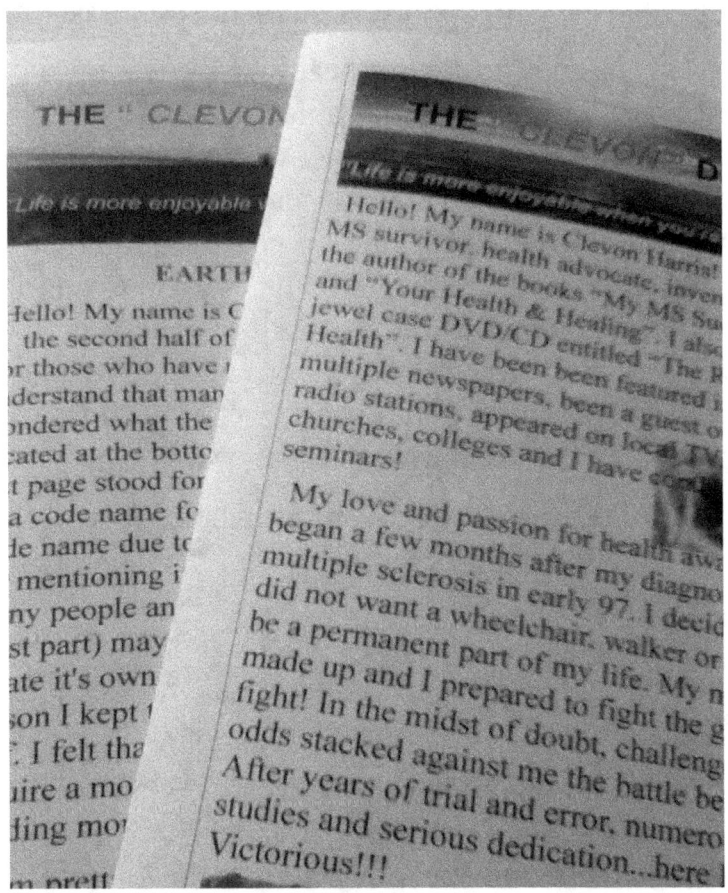

3 tbsp of the Red Star nutritional yeast brand had:

B12 1000% Thiamin 830% Riboflavin 780% B6 680%

THE "CLEVON" DIET

My name is Clevon Harris. I am a MS survivor, health advocate, inventor and author of *My MS Success*, *Your Health And Healing* and *Suffering With A Smile*. My jewel case DVD/CD *The Road To Health* stresses the importance of a healthy diet and a clean colon. I have been featured in multiple newspapers, been a guest on several radio stations, appeared on local TV, spoke at churches, colleges and I have been a speaker at numerous seminars.

My love and passion for health awareness began a few months after my multiple sclerosis diagnosis in early 97. I decided I did not want a wheelchair, walker or cane to be a permanent part of my life. My mind was made up and I prepared to fight the good fight. In the midst of doubt, challenges and odds stacked against me the battle began. After years of trial, error, fasting, numerous studies and serious dedication, here I stand; victorious. I try to consume a 20% acidity/80% alkaline diet daily.

I had a remarkable recovery from being disabled. For more than 13 years; I worked a standing job in the heat, no medication, no fatigue, 7-9 hour shifts, and had plenty of energy as I clocked out. I kept on improving. Carnitine helps aid muscle reflexes. Eat carnitine with carbohydrates for proper absorption.

I have been asked by many people, "What is your diet?" and "What did you do?" In this brochure, I am pleased to inform you. The "Clevon" diet may be a diet in theory but in reality it is a process. It's time to reclaim what you once had.

The "Clevon" diet consists of the **CED** process. This process has the potential to help not only MS patients but many other patients with other serious ailments as well. You may ask the question "What is **CED**?" Well, let's get started.

C = Colon (*Calcium pg 53, *Collagen)

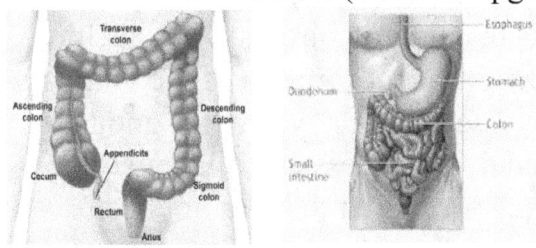

Nourish and clean your colon. I have read it and you may have heard it. Your life and death depend a lot upon the health of your colon. The quality of the food you eat is vital and very important to your daily life. Proper nutrition rebuilds and regenerates the cells and tissues of our body. It's best when our bodies are properly nourished consistently. Excess fried, overcooked or processed foods along with excess sugar or excess salt could cause starvation of the colon and cause damage to muscles, nerves, cells and tissues of the walls of the colon. If your colon is unclean, it will affect your whole body. Reclaiming optimal health can be difficult or next to impossible to achieve if you have an unclean colon and /or low intestinal flora. Prior to my MS diagnosis, I was eating very few healthy foods and to many unhealthy foods. I had to change my diet.

Any toxins, waste matter and feces should all be eliminated from our bodies. Water, salt, dark leafy greens, fiber and herbal teas help clean our colon.

When we consume raw foods high in fiber and roughage, keep in mind that they are helping clean the large and small intestines out by naturally pushing (or sweeping) the decaying waste through the interior walls. Walls of the intestines become covered with a mucus plaque due to our bodies naturally trying to block unsafe toxins from entering our bloodstream. Over a period of time this mucus gets thicker upon eating poorly. Intestinal walls that are too dirty, are not healthy enough to allow proper absorption of the vitamins and minerals we need in our system for good health. Deficiencies, sickness and ailments follow afterwords. Imagine a toilet that has not been flushed or if the garbage man stops running. That would be very unhealthy and it would definitely cause problems. Even the very best diets on Earth would do little help for us if our colon is clogged with waste matter. We need to nourish and clean our colon. We can have our colon cleansed by a healthy fast or a process called Colon Irrigation. Water is used to blast and knock the fecal matter loose. Make sure that your operator is certified. This procedure may take more than one visit depending upon how much waste matter you have accumulated. We all eat differently so our accumulation of waste will vary. Enemas and colon cleanse pills are not nearly as effective as fasting or a colon irrigation cleanse in my opinion. Based upon the colon cleanse that I had, it was very safe and there was nothing to worry about. I had my cleanse recorded for educational purposes. I reached my cecum release and it can be seen on my DVD "The Road To Health". Many people made the decision to get a colon cleanse after viewing my cleanse. For more info or booking search for colonic or colon irrigation in your area.

E = Enzymes (*Exercise: Boost Dopamine)

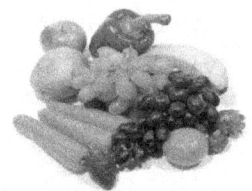

Load your body with enzymes. After cleaning your colon, continue putting healthy live foods in your system. In order to best obtain enzymes, eat uncooked, unprocessed fruit, vegetables and foods asap after buying. Most leafy green vegetables lose nutrients very quickly in our refrigerators due to no light. Enzymes are used for body repair, they are anti-aging and give us energy. I believe many MS patients quickly fatigue and get weak from heat due to them not having enough enzymes stored in their bodies. Heat (an enemy of MS) will destroy enzymes depending on the temperature or method. Low enzymes result in illness, fast aging and poor health. An enzyme rich diet can give us a stronger *immune system* and the potentiality to recover from sicknesses at a higher rate than a diet poor in them. Pineapple, papaya, mango and raw honey are some top sources. Vegetables are high in silica (pg 163).

Another great way to help your body create new cells and boundless energy after a colon cleanse is to consume marine phytoplankton. What is it? Phyton = plant   Planktos = wandering

Marine Phytoplankton

Humpback Whales

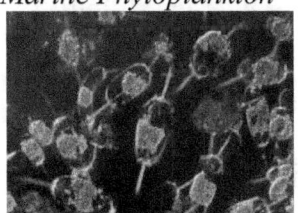

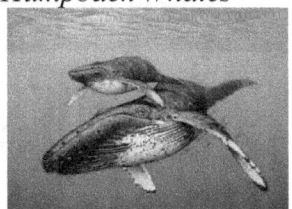

Phytoplankton is the food whales have lived on for many years, is responsible for up to 90% of the earth's oxygen and can increase oxygen uptake. It is earth's first nutrient dense super food and it contains naturally produced vitamins and minerals. It has 400 times the energy of any known plant. It has the ability to give you short and long term energy so you can feel energy now as well as have some left over in your reservoir for later. I have tried Phytoplankton. It did not have a bad taste and I could feel positive results. Many people have not heard of this plant. If this plant is new to you, you can look it up online to learn more about it as well as purchase some for consumption. This plant food is what whales feed on daily to keep them healthy and living for a long time. If it helps them, surely it can benefit us. **Fulvic Acid Mineral Complex** is another product I highly recommend. I drink fulvic to expel harmful metallic minerals and toxins from my body. Silica (page 163) is found in fulvic.

D = Diet (Monitor Diet, *Vitamin D)

Quality **Protein** (whey, chicken, fish) with BCAA in your diet is essential for providing solid muscle, strength, endurance, immunity, bone strength and transporting numerous necessities like hormones, DNA, oxygen, etc throughout your body. Vitamin **K** is a necessity. It is essential for proper brain and nervous function and it will significantly fight any inflammation within the body. K will need healthy **dietary fat** to absorb. Dietary fats improve vitamin and mineral absorption (40% of our body is protein). **Beans** provide a lot of benefits. Make sure they are consumed often. Eat clams and salt in moderation.

Remembering The Four Food Groups

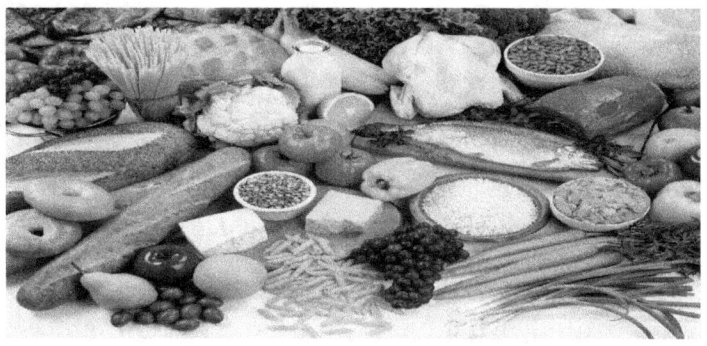

Many people have left their nutritional values of eating a well balanced meal daily and have decided to lean towards the fast food life. When monitoring your diet, be sure you consume healthy portions of each one of the four food groups on a daily basis. Consuming the foods together as a group, will help many vitamins and minerals perform at their best. Some foods need the assistance of other foods just as vitamin K needs dietary fat to absorb. Eating the four food groups together is ideal, eating each food group separate could help generate certain nutrient deficiencies. In the photo above you see a ham but I rarely include pork in my diet. The human body does not digest pork as easy as it does fish, chicken or turkey (my 3 most consistent meats). Romaine, iceberg and spinach are the leafy green vegetables I prefer. The salad dressing helps our body absorb vitamins and minerals. (I like **miso soup** 3x a day.)

Genesis 1: 29 *And God said, Behold I have given you every herb bearing seed, which is upon the face of all the earth, and every tree, in the which is the fruit of a tree yielding seed; to you it shall be for meat.* (I eat **lycopene** rich food often. Pg 102)

Ezekiel 47: 12 -- *and the fruit thereof shall be meat, and the leaf thereof for medicine.*

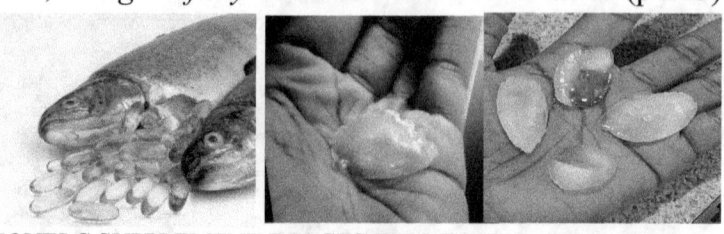

NOVELC SUPPLEMENT IMAGES WILL DIFFER. **5 Vons above.**

For healthier results, I prefer my fish, chicken or steaks broiled. All fish are not equal in Omega-3s. In my book *Your Health And Healing*, I explained the difference. Omega-3 pills that turn cloudy in the freezer aren't quality. Quality pills will not turn cloudy/freeze. Fish provide vitamin D and iodine.

Deuteronomy 14:9 *These ye shall eat of all that are in the waters: all that have fins and scales shall ye eat:* Verse 10 says *And whatsoever hath not fins and scales ye may not eat; it is unclean unto you.* Also read Leviticus 11:9, 10, 11 and 12 for more information on clean and unclean meats.

Jesus fed the multitude two fish and five loaves in Math: 14:19. I am pretty sure Jesus would not eat or offer harmful food. Jesus was given fish to eat in the book of Luke.

Luke 24:42 *And they gave him a piece of a broiled fish, and of an honeycomb.* Verse 43 says *And he took it, and did eat before them.*

Myoglobin is the iron and oxygen protein I later discovered from eating steak in the late 90s. Many believe the red liquid is blood but it isn't. (*see page 123*). I also eat red tuna for myoglobin. Red tuna is healthier and easier to digest than steaks. If I take a *fish collagen,* it will be from cod, snapper or tilapia (***found in most marine collagen***). I will never ingest shellfish, jellyfish or shark collagen knowingly.

Seaweed Salad *Smoothies* *Sushi*

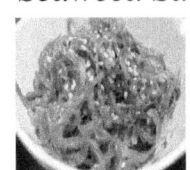 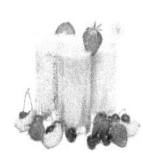 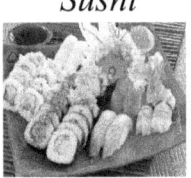

Eating healthy does not have to be boring. There are a plethora of foods and various ways to prepare them. I eat seaweed salad because I enjoy the taste, iodine content and the health and healing benefits of Wakame seaweed. I eat Nori seaweed a lot. It is used to wrap sushi. Spirulina algae is also healthy. Smoothies and vanilla bean ice cream are eaten as a healthy treat. Cheese (*whey*), avocado, rice, nuts, whole grains and berries give me energy. I often drink almond milk and plenty of water (60-70% of our body is water). Fatigue, heart attack, headache, lower back pain, bladder cancer, cholesterol, joint pain and blood pressure can be fought by drinking water (I always add water to my Isopure). **CED** is able to fight **"many"** ailments, help people lose unwanted weight and assist in reclaiming health.

Sometimes I'll cheat and eat something unhealthy like pizza or a hamburger but I do it moderately. I let my healthy eating outweigh unhealthy eating by a large margin. No one wants to struggle or depend on others for balance. No one wants a setback after overcoming adversity. I eat various fermented food and cheese (for calcium, pg 53). I try to exercise and sweat daily to achieve healthy blood sugar levels.

Always remember that the words *"no cure"* does not mean that you will never get well. Knowledge is power. Let's reign over sickness. Never give up on your dreams! **"Life is more enjoyable when you're healthy!"** ~ **Clevon Harris**

MAKE THE *"CLEVON"* DIET AND **CED** PART OF YOUR HEALTHY LIFESTYLE TODAY!!!

1. We need hydrochloric acid in the stomach to aid in proper digestion, absorption and better health.

2. Consume probiotics & feed them with prebiotics to increase healthy intestinal flora. (pg 206)

*3. Eat **enzyme/alkaline/anti-inflammatory** foods.*

4. Eat healthy, drink plenty of water and exercise.

5. Sweating detoxifies our body, reduces stress and strengthens our heart and immune system.

6. Sphingolipids, myoglobin, magnesium, vitamins D and K, iron, selenium and tyrosine are in tuna.

7. Red meat is #1 in carnitine which assists muscle movement etc. Carnosine aids immune system etc.

8. Eat red meat moderately. Milk is #3 in carnitine.

9. Skim milk has more carnitine than whole milk.

10. Concentrated **whey protein** has **prime** carnitine levels.

Amazon.com/author/clevonharris **OR** Fightingsickness.com

For more information: Miracleintentions@yahoo.com

Clevon Harris

THE " CLEVON " DIET

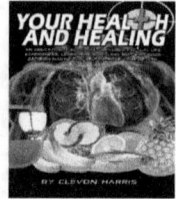
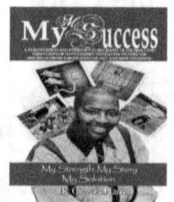
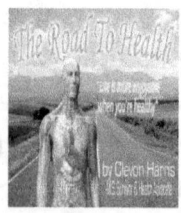

THE " CLEVON " DIET

"Life is more enjoyable when you're healthy!"

EARTH RED

Hello! My name is Clevon Harris. Welcome to the second half of THE"CLEVON" DIET. For those who have read the first half, I understand that many people have seen and wondered what the words EARH RED located at the bottom right hand corner of the last page stood for. Those words were written as a code name for red dirt. I wrote it as a code name due to the fact that my purpose for mentioning it is seemingly unheard of by many people and the information (for the most part) may raise many questions and create it's own share of doubters. For that reason I kept the first half separate from this half. I felt that explaining Earth Red would require a more in depth approach, therefore needing more of it's own personal space.

I am sure there will be some people that question my thoughts and there will be some who will understand my thoughts and what I am saying. While I do practice the process mentioned in this half of the diet. It **"is"** optional and it does not have to be combined with the first half of THE "CLEVON" DIET to achieve results. The first half is my signature, this half is basically food for thought. The choice is totally up to the individual.

Why did I practice this process? What made me think of this? Why am I sharing this information? These questions and much more will be answered shortly. It's time to reclaim what you once had.

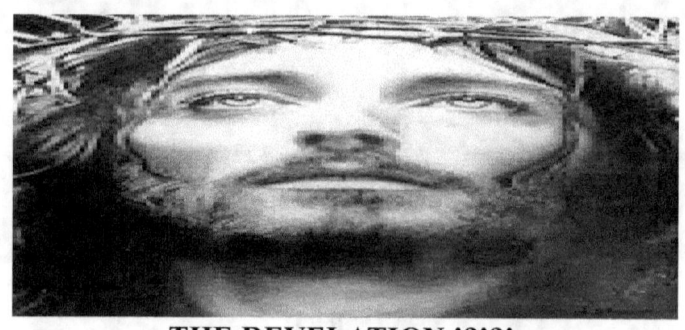

THE REVELATION !?!?!

I was visiting a local church. Bible study had just ended and the pastor asked if he could have a word with me in private. The pastor knows that I am a health advocate and he wanted to share with me a revelation that had been revealed to him during prayer and meditation. He told me that he asked God something on the lines of, "With so many people being diagnosed with cancer, MS and all of these diseases and ailments at such a fast pace, what should we do?"

The pastor said the answer was ***"Eat some red dirt!"***

The pastor said that if we think about it, God formed us from dirt. He mentioned Genesis 2:7 which says *And the Lord God formed man of the dust of the ground, and breathed into his nostrils the breath of life; and man became a living soul.* I agreed with him and we both referenced the end verse of Genesis 3:19 which says *for dust thou art, and unto dust shalt thou return.* The pastor explained that you can't eat just any dirt. The soil needs to be clean with no chemicals or anything sprayed on it. He also stated that you should not get the dirt from the very top. The dirt should be dug and gathered from further underneath the ground. I asked him how much should a person consume and how often. He replied "not a lot". He said that only a sprinkle or "pinch" twice a month should be effective. I want to say he emphasized the **pinch size** amount. Either way, it was not a large amount to be consumed twice a month.

At first I was kinda taken by surprise by the pastor's revelation. However this was not my first time hearing something like this. Previously in 2003, I had read a real life story on how a very ill stricken man gained his health back by eating some dirt to aid him in his recovery. This guy did not specify how to retrieve the dirt or what kind to eat but he did say eat "a little" dirt. At first glance, I thought this guy was crazy! I did not think to much more about this guy or his book until years later in late 2007 after the Pastor shared his revelation with me.

Days later I was explaining the pastor's revelation with this young white lady I know. She looked very surprised and said "It makes sense now!" I asked her to explain what she meant! She told me that on her way back home from a fellowship trip with some of her female friends they stopped at the gas station. She said around two or three of her black friends got off the bus and went to some red dirt and began digging. She said they began to eat some of the dirt and she thought they were crazy. One of the girls said it helped with her asthma and another said she was anemic. They said if you do it, make sure to dig and get your dirt from under the soil and not off the top. Coming from people that had never met one another before, their stories sounded all to similar to me.

A few weeks later I began to consume a **pinch size** amount of red dirt twice a month. I even tried putting some of the dirt in capsules in hopes of achieving better absorption. I wondered what vitamins, minerals or what was found in this dirt. With my health already in good shape, I wondered if it was even helping me any. I did this for only about three months. I began to lose the motivation I had and I eventually discontinued the pinch size red dirt process.

MY REVELATION!?!?!

As you know, a clean colon is the first step in The "CLEVON" Diet. I consumed healthy foods that nourished and helped clean my colon on a regular basis for so long that I reached my cecum release during my first colon irrigation cleanse back in 2005(The Road To Health DVD). A healthy diet is great but sometimes you may need some help from an irrigation cleanse depending upon how much unhealthy foods you have consumed over time. I continued to practice the **CED** process and inform others how important it is.

In late 2013, as I was in deep meditation. I asked God why did I feel such a close connection with the pastor's revelation many years ago? What, if anything is beneficial in the dirt? Why did I believe and feel so strongly that there was something there but nothing ever materialized? The answer did not come that day. The answer did not even come that night. One night as I prepared to take a nap and get some rest, out of nowhere a bright light and question hit me!

"The red dirt may help clean your colon?"

All of a sudden I could not sleep. I got up and was not tired anymore. My mind could not see anything but people being healed and reclaiming their health. I actually got really excited! This was one of my desires and dreams. This will be a blessing to many!

Colon Irrigation Procedure

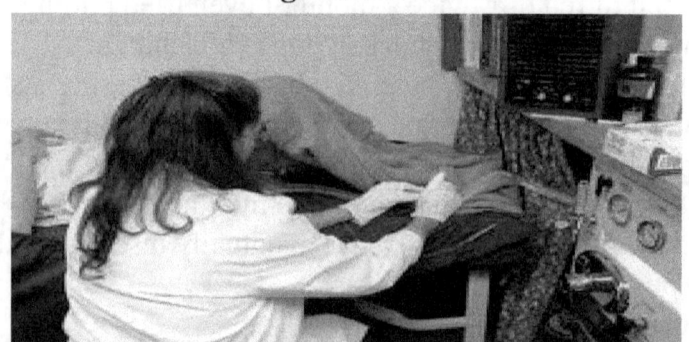

The following days I began to do more studies on red dirt. I began the consumption of it twice a month again. I stay regular and it never constipates me. As a MS survivor, I did notice that the desire to stretch from feeling stiff as I stood up had shortened. That feels great! I had far less cramps in my feet than I previously had. Sometimes I was so accustom to the cramps, stretching and feeling stiff to a point where it had become normal to me. I believe that the vitamins and minerals found in the foods I was consuming were being absorbed into my system a lot better with the help of the red dirt helping to clean my colon by pushing unwanted fecal matter out. Even though I eat healthy, just a **"little bit"** of unhealthy food consumed isn't good for the colon. It adds up and some of it is often left behind. It needs to be removed and expelled from the body.

I had a chance to sit down and talk to a 94 year old cousin of mine. We talked and discussed many things but as you know, we eventually ended up discussing people eating red dirt. There was not a lot of information I gathered from her but she said that her mother (or grandmother) use to put a pan of it in the oven and bake it. The reason was to dry it out, if it was wet and sloppy. My cousin said that she does not know specifically what it was good for but she just knew it was good for you. She said that she would often crave it. I decided to go online to get a better understanding on why other people would consume red dirt. This is what I found.

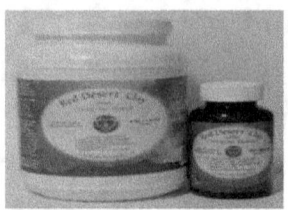 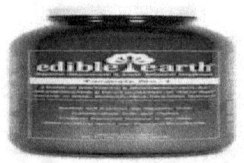

Iron is a very very common element in soils. When oxidized, iron forms reddish colored minerals (basically rust and similar compounds)

1. Geophagia is the practice of eating dirt, especially clay like soils, which is something animals and people have been doing for ages.

2. People eat dirt to satisfy a physiological need for iron or other nutrients lacking from individuals' diet.

3. There is a slight chance it could help develop the immune system.

4. Even in humans there are few reports of infections routinely associated with geophagy by pregnant women in sub-Saharan Africa, probably because women take clays from 60 cm to 90 cm below the soil surface and at least some of the time they bake the clay before consuming.

5. In the Yazoo Mississippi Delta, Negroes and whites send requests to their upcountry friends for a bit of red clay, declaring that black Delta soil is "right bad eating." In certain parts of Mississippi, poor whites will walk miles for a spoonful of dirt from a favorite bank of clay because it "tastes sour, like a lemon." In other sections of the South, some top their meals with a savory tablespoon of dirt.

6. A lot of pregnant women eat dirt because of the minerals such as calcium, sodium and iron which support energy production and other vital biological processes because it has minerals and they just get a craving for it. Those who aren't pregnant say they like the earthy taste.

7. Specific soils [may be] serving to cleanse and De-worm consumer's intestinal tracts.

MY OPINION AND MY BELIEF!

I believe if we would eat healthy, the very foods we consume would allow our colon to remain clean. Once we began to eat unhealthy foods, our colon begins to need help eliminating the accumulated fecal matter. I believe that red dirt will help push and clean it out. A colon irrigation is the best way to clean your colon in my opinion. I was told put a teaspoon of red dirt in 8oz of water & soak for about 30 min. Water will become a detox medicine. I prefer a pinch of dirt over the water.

Who will this diet benefit? I believe The "Clevon" Diet will benefit many people suffering from various health ailments. Why red dirt? I believe the other soils may potentially interfere with the absorption rate of certain vitamins and minerals and the texture is not as durable or equipped for the cause. Since red dirt was specified, I used a pinch of red dirt + 1 tbsp of ACV.

Psalm 103:14 *For he knoweth our frame; he remembereth that we are dust.*

You may have heard there is nothing new under the sun! What about under your feet? Always remember that the words *"no cure"* does not mean that you will never get well. Never give up on your dreams! Let's reign over sickness! Knowledge is power! **"Life is more enjoyable when you're healthy!"** ~ Clevon Harris

Amazon.com/author/clevonharris **OR** Fightingsickness.com

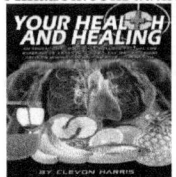 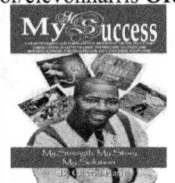 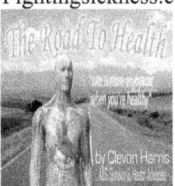

For more information: Miracleintentions@yahoo.com

MIRACLES DO HAPPEN

There may be times when we feel as if all is lost and there is nothing else we can do. My advice to you is to never give up and always believe. There is no medicine like hope and "trusting" in almighty God. Our God is awesome!!! Miracles do happen!

1. People that suffer from epilepsy may need to try adding manganese to their diet.

2. Behavior problems, aggressive tendencies, mean violent behavior or mental instability problems can possibility be toned down by adding the minerals chromium, copper, vanadium or lithium to the diet.

3. Chromium, vanadium and lithium are all helpful in the treatment of Attention Deficit Disorders also known as ADD.

THE HEALTHY GREEN POWDERS I PREFER
(I usually combine with purified or distilled water.)
For a healthy, alkalized, energy filled body, you can achieve that goal by consuming a quality green drink. I've tried and recommend using Vitamineral Greens TM by Health Force TM , Green Vibrance by Vibrant Health and Athletic Greens by Athletic Greens. All are great products and were mentioned as the top 3 green drinks available on the market at the time of my latest research. Many diseases and serious ailments cannot live in an alkaline/oxygen rich environment like these 3 products can provide. Many powders are best consumed in the morning.

MIRACLES DO HAPPEN

I mentioned within this publication that there are certain foods if we combine and eat them together, they can provide our body with even better health results than if we were to eat them alone. Broccoli + tomatoes, olive oil + turmeric + pepper, garlic + citrus fruits or eating oatmeal with orange juice are just a few combinations. Although I did not write a chapter on beans, I did eat Navy and pinto beans prior to both of my MS victories. They can prevent heart disease, fight cancer, lower cholesterol, help you lose weight and help manage diabetes. Beans are packed with protein, fiber, B-vitamins, iron and potassium but they do have their health risk factors as well. Beans can raise blood pressure, interfere with vitamin absorption, cause headaches, trigger gout and make some people gassy. Again, I did eat beans but not a whole lot. Beans were not one of my main recovery foods I used to assist me during this last MS setback. The *avocado fruit* (which are used to make *guacamole*) does not have it's own chapter either. However, I have and continue to use it in my salads (*see page 38*). Avocados have more potassium than a banana, fights breast and prostate cancer and helps lower cholesterol. Not to mention it also fights arthritis, helps support cardiovascular and eye health and it has the vitamin K that I seek. *Avocados help the body better absorb important nutrients and increases the nutrient value of plant foods you are consuming.* Avocado is the best fruit source for vitamin E. Avocados provide protection from strokes due to the rich *myelin repairing folate* (aka B9) it has. This fruit has plenty of it.

Cinnamon has been used since Biblical times due to it's sweet scent and medicinal purposes. Honey has a number of health benefits when consumed by itself as well. As I mentioned earlier, some foods become more powerful and potent once they are combined with certain foods. Honey + cinnamon is another prime example of that. Both contain water, protein, fiber, sugars and numerous vitamins and minerals. They also contain the minerals calcium, copper, iron, manganese, magnesium, phosphorus, potassium, selenium, sodium and zinc. They also contain the vitamins B-6, vitamin C, folate, niacin and riboflavin. Cinnamon carries the fat soluble vitamins A, E and K. One teaspoon of cinnamon a day or just two cinnamon sticks is a reasonable amount. I will often add cinnamon and/or honey to my protein shakes. The list on page 193 will show you benefits that cinnamon can assist you with by itself. A star next to the health benefit just means if honey is combined with the cinnamon, that benefit will be enhanced. Cinnamon can be used for...

Anti-oxidant - Cinnamon has an ORAC value of 267,536 umol TE/100g (100 grams or about 3.5 ounces). It is one of the top 7 anti-oxidants in the world. It can greatly lower the risk of disease.

Candida Yeast Infections – Cinnamon tea infused with cinnamon leaf or Bark oil shows an amazing ability to stop medication resistant yeast infections. (I eat apples + cinnamon and drink green tea + honey.)

Weight Loss – Curves appetite, speeds metabolism

(Do not mix cinnamon with blood thinning medications because cinnamon also has a blood thinning effect.)

MIRACLES DO HAPPEN

*Stronger Immune System

*Reduce hair loss and stimulate hair growth

*Skin care (If mixed into a paste, it can fight acne, wrinkles and bites.)

*Digestion

*Cancer

*Arthritis/Osteoporosis (Bones need manganese.)

*Heart Health

*Lowering LDL cholesterol and triglycerides

*Tooth Decay, Tooth Aches and Gum Disease

*Type 2 Diabetes/Blood Sugar Control

Stomach Bug/Flu

Irritable Bowel Syndrome (IBS)

Anti-Bacterial/Anti-Microbial/Toenail Fungus

Food Preservative

Odor Neutralizer

Can relieve muscle pain

Can help memory, alertness or calm nerves

Helps PMS

Attention Deficit Disorder

Alzheimer's Disease

Parkinson's Disease

Fight Salmonella and E.coli

Virus Fighter: Cold, Cough, Sore Throat

Mood Enhancer/Reduced Irritability

Red Dirt (This method is not for everyone)

I tried using one teaspoon of red dirt and I let it soak in a full glass of water for thirty minutes. To my understanding, several hours is preferable. The water activates its electromagnetic charge. Be sure to remove the metallic spoon used to stir from the water. The longer the clay soaks in the water the more it imparts its electromagnetic charge into the water, making the water into medicine. The whole glass gets charged, so *you don't need very much of the physical red dirt/clay itself* to draw toxins. Red dirt water should be ingested on an empty stomach early in the morning or before bed. Drink plenty of water throughout the day. A daily regime can be as long as three weeks, then you should break from it for at least a week. Avoid combining red dirt water with pharmaceutical or homeopathic medicines. It is best to make sure that you are clear of any type medicine regime before trying red dirt water. The action of the red dirt is inhibited by medicines. Red dirt can absorb harmful toxins from the body. I use 1 tbsp of ACV with a pinch of red dirt to absorb silica.

Stiffness And Constantly Stretching

Inflammation and water retention in the body can result from consuming excessive unhealthy acidic foods. This can put pressure on your nerves and can lead to joint pain and stiffness. Anything that is poison to our bodies should be eliminated because toxins in our body lead to stress. An abundance of toxins in the body can cause muscles to tighten and spasm. Nonprescription medication, coffee, MSG, alcohol, fast food, soda,to much dairy products and chocolate need to be avoided. Consume calcium-rich foods such as yogurt, omega-3 fatty acids (fish such as mackerel or salmon), calcium supplements, a plethora of vegetables, leafy greens (like spinach, kale), figs, broccoli and parsley. For better health results add tomatoes and lettuce to your hamburger and/or chicken sandwiches. Instead of eating fried french fries, try substituting them with a side salad.

Exercise improves muscle strength, increase joint flexibility, endurance and can relieve symptoms of stress, depression and anxiety. It can decrease your risk of stroke, colon cancer, heart disease, diabetes and high blood pressure. Moderate activities such as walking, swimming, biking or even organized sports contribute to your physical fitness needs. It is best to warm up for 5 to 10 minutes to increase your blood flow and prepare your body for activity. This will help reduce any risk of injury.

Note: *Oregano can counter slight spasms. Pickle juice (Dill) fights cramps, promotes healthy flora. Coconut water or turmeric can also fight cramps.*

Plantar Wart (page 111 #18, bottom of page 200.)

Many people have plantar warts on the bottom of their feet but have no clue on what to do to get rid of them. I had three plantar warts on my feet for more than ten years. One wart was on the bottom of one of my small toes. I had two bigger plantar warts on the balls of each of my feet. When I was walking, every step that I took was pretty painful. Many people suggested that I have them surgically removed. If possible, I definitely was not wanting any type of surgery. Having them removed or cut out is not only extra money to spend but it would have lead to unwanted missed days away from my job due to recovery time for my feet. The first time I developed the plantar warts, I purchased several products to destroy them but they all failed.

I later found and purchased a foot soak from a supermarket that contained a minimal amount of **dead sea** salt (*not to be confused with sea salt*) in it. In less than two weeks the wart and pain started to fade away. Since my foot was healing at such a fast pace, I neglected to buy another pack of the foot soak. I assumed that the wart would continue to fade away on its on. As time went by, the wart began to slowly come back. After returning to the supermarket to purchase the same exact product, I was informed they no longer carried it. So, it was back to the drawing board as I began searching for an alternative. The Epsom salt I purchased did not help my feet one bit. Salicylic acid and many other products I purchased began to fall short as well.

I was at a lady's yard sale and because I was one of her regulars, she observed as I walked my feet were obviously bothering me that day. I explained to her what was going on and she told me a story about how her son had recently suffered from the same problem. She said as he was vacationing at the beach in Florida, he spent a lot of time in the water. To both her and her son's surprise, the water appeared to be healing his feet. She said it was like nothing she had ever seen before. "It was as if the water was slowly pulling the warts out of his feet" she said. Her son informed her later that he did not suffer any discomfort during his healing process.

After hearing about her son's success story with him soaking either in the ocean or sea, I thought about the success I once enjoyed due to soaking in a dead sea salt soak. I later purchased dead sea salt online. I had finally found what I was looking for and at a remarkable price. After applying a reliable foot repair cream to the wart, I add dead sea salt to that area. The salt will stick to the cream and both can be taped and easily held secure. It took a few days to feel and notice a difference but my walk improved and it began to look normal again. I wish I could find a product with this already combined. I also mix 3-4 drops of **oregano oil** with 1 tsp of a **carrier oil** like **neem oil**. I swab the wart with this mixture and tape it 4-5 times a day. I like it. I also use **black tar salve**. It can help draw plantar seeds out. Put a small amount on the area and cover/tape it 2-3 times a day for 3-4 weeks. (I use **duct** tape.)

Garlic Lodged In Throat

I used garlic salt on a regular basis during my first year of my MS diagnosis but I later changed over to garlic powder. In late 2014, I became very interested in the many beneficial health properties of raw garlic. I then decided to change over to raw chopped garlic. I did not want to go through the process of chewing it so I tried to take a shortcut. I took two garlic cloves and cut them into smaller pieces with a knife. My plan was to swallow the small pieces in the same manner I would swallow my vitamins. Unfortunately it did not work out that way for me. As I attempted to swallow one of the pieces, obviously I did not cut it small enough. It appeared to fall to the left side of my throat and then it became lodged there. After two days of wheezing while breathing, constantly smelling the garlic and knowing that it was still lodged in my throat, I became frustrated and concerned. Other people could easily hear wheezing. My breathing sounded very similar to a person suffering from bronchitis.

All my attempts to dislodge the garlic appeared to be useless & in vain. I checked myself into the ER where they did an X-ray. They saw exactly where the garlic was lodged and basically told me that it would be best to try letting it pass on it's on. If it had not passed in the next two days, I was asked to return. I went home and prayed about the situation. I asked God for his guidance because I definitely did not want to go back to the hospital. As I went to sleep that night, I had a strange dream. I was at a restaurant eating with someone and as I prepared to leave, I decided to purchase four canned sodas. While checking out, I saw that I had two different flavors. I exited the restaurant, the dream came to an end and I woke up.

I woke up the next morning wondering why I had a dream about buying four sodas. I might drink a small amount of soda every now and then but soda is clearly not a part of my staying healthy lifestyle. I decided to just dismiss the dream as not really having any significant value. Later that day I was on the internet searching for helpful alternatives to *"getting food dislodged from the throat"*. While I browsed, I was observant and watchful of anything that could possibly be God leading me. I soon ran across this particular Q&A forum.....

"""I once had food lodged in my throat before.

I've been sick since last week and my throat is swollen. I was eating raw garlic on a slice of sprouted bread w/some olive oil and after I ate that I felt like there was something stuck in my throat. It's still there today and I have an appointment w/an ear, nose, and throat specialist tomorrow. The doctor today diagnosed me w/larnygitis. I had a steroid shot only because we hope it may reduce the swelling in my throat and help the food become dislodged. So far it hasn't done that.

Does anyone know how I can get this thing unstuck myself? It really hurts!
Thanks!!

littlefamily said
> *This happened to my Mom and she went into the emergency room. They gave her soda pop (I'm pretty sure just regular coke). There is something in it that is supposed to make the throat get a bit larger and the food can go down.*
>
> *It worked for her.*
>
> *Hope you are already doing better.*

I'm the same as earlier. I'm drinking a Coke right now! Thanks!"""

After reading this, I immediately thought back to the dream I had. I then drove to the closest store to purchase four canned cokes. They were sold out of canned cokes that day so I decided to buy two, 2 liter cokes. I would need to drink four 12 oz cups of coke to match the dream. Upon returning home I was excited! I was believing that God was talking to me through the dream. I drank one 12 oz cup, then another about an hour later. I drank the third 12 oz cup of coke about another hour after that. Nothing happened! I had one more 12 oz of soda to drink to match the four canned drinks I saw in the dream. I was now both nervous and hesitant to drink the fourth 12 oz cup because I had become worried that God was possibly not talking to me through the dream. If God was not leading me, I was not ready to accept it.

Later that night I was in my room typing and my brother went to the refrigerator. I heard the sound of a carbonated drink being opened. As he passed by me, I noticed that he was drinking some orange soda. Could this be the reason I saw two flavors in the dream? I got up, went to the kitchen and filled the fourth and final 12 oz cup with the orange soda this time. In less than 5 minutes, I uncontrollably began coughing. A lot of thick mucus was forced out along with the garlic. Surprisingly, the garlic still looked freshly cut! I was relieved, very happy and the wheezing was all gone. I kept praising God and thanking Jesus! **Miracles do happen!**
(**Note: Duct** tape can suffocate/kill a wart...Pg 197, or tape ACV cotton ball on wart nightly till it dies.)

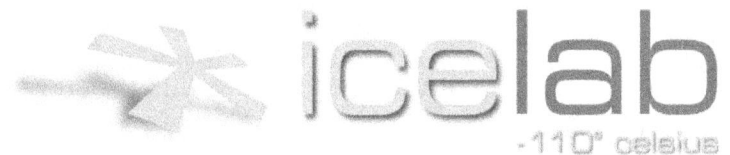

Years ago when playing sports, our coach would have us relax in a big tub of ice for more than 20 minutes. We now have Cryotherapy (cold sauna) invented by Professor Toshiro Yamauchi in 1980. Many professional athletes today step into cold saunas to heal their bodies. Hot saunas have plus 110c and cold saunas minus 110c. No one shivers in the cold sauna because the climate is dry and not wet. You will inhale a lot of oxygen and only 2 to 3 minutes a day is needed to get health benefits. If soaking in a bath tub full of ice healed many injuries, sprains and shin splints we athletes had years ago, I am confident this new technology will provide the same and better results just in a more modern and convenient manner. This stand up Ice Lab can treat pinched nerves, arthritis, cellulite, ect and possibly help MS sufferers by helping the nervous system. Also see **CryoTherapyMiami**.

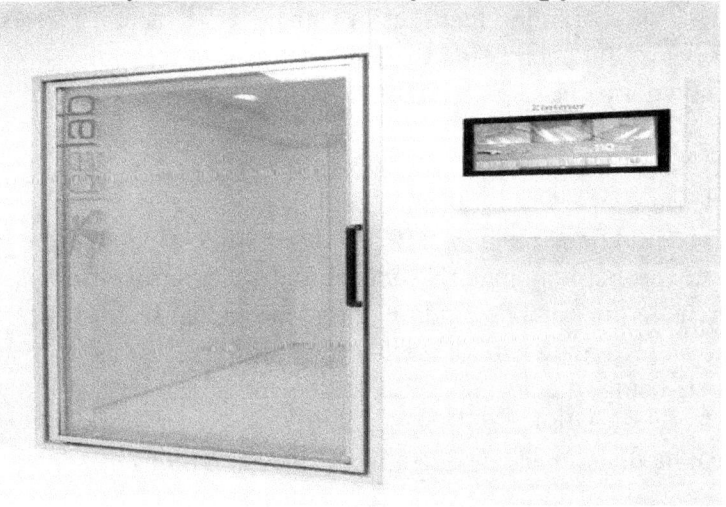

If you have questions in regards to this procedure, contact information is available ahead thanks to the informative e-mail I received from Mr. Rainer Bolsinger. Research this *adrenaline* sauna today!

icelab-inSports:
Pre-cooling: increase performance, power and endurance
Intermediate cooling: optimise training, by shortening break between training units
Post-colling: faster recovery and reduction/skipping of bad effects of exhausting training or competition.
Pain control, stress management, sports medicine and rehabilitation
Leisure: running, cycling, climbing, diving, surfing, skiing...
Fitness: integrate in workout, performance, agility, slimming... program

Some references: INSEP/Paris (all sports), Bundesleistungszentrum Kienbaum (training centre of 7 national sports associations and federal police), National training facilities of the French Rugby Federation (FFR), FC Bayer Leverkusen, Rolland Garros (One of the 4 Grand Slam tournaments), FC Porto, Nad Al Sheba Club (Exclusive training facilities in Dubai), FC Krasnor, FC Bayern München ... many more and many more well known top class sports facilities will follow!

icelab-inSpa:
Please visit www.cold-sauna.com
The Cold Sauna icelab -110 °C in Spa is a real multi-fitter and is capable to make a connection between the different areas in the hotel depending on the individual focus of each house. No matter if the orientation is towards business, well-being, medical spa, fitness, leisure, adventure & lifestyle, beauty ... with icelab in many cases a fruitful fit can be developed. Beside it is an attraction by itself!

ICE-LAB

General use: As a spa day starter. A welcome Jet-Lag treatment. The intermediate Di-Stress, sleep well or charge your battery offer. ...

... Focused use: as part of programs: sports, fitness, beauty, leisure, preventive health, indication orientated, ...

Some references:

Monaco: Thermes Marins www.thermesmarinsmontecarlo.com (luxury, casino, wellbeing...)

Canada: Sparkling Hill Resort: www.sparklinghill.com (luxury, curative)

Austria / Germany: www.kurzentrum.com (9 sites, 9 x icelab: medical and welness)

Czech Republic: Carlsbad Plaza's Carlsbad Clinic

Turkey: Gloria Sports Hotel (sports, fitness...)

Russia: Radisson Sochi

China: Evergrande Tjian Jin (placed in aesthetic clinic related to sports centre, casino, 5* hotel...)

Azerbaijan coming soon: Gabala Lake Palace with Chenot Spa (luxury, health, detox, ...)

We stood out with 3 diamonds at the European Health & Spa Award in Vienna:https://www.flickr.com/photos/bestevent_pictures/18924191256/in/album-72157652436362724/

If you would like any further information, please let me know.

Warmest regards and a nice day!

Rainer

Rainer Bolsinger
Zimmer MedizinSysteme GmbH
Junkersstraße 9
D-89231 Neu-Ulm
Germany
Tel + 49 731 9761 - 198
Mobil + 49 1520 90 97 922
Fax + 49 731 9761 - 118
eMail r.bolsinger@zimmer.de
Internet www.zimmer.de // icelab-M

Back when I was in school, we constantly studied the importance of consuming the four food groups. Meat, milk, bread/grains and the fruit & vegetable group. Our school lunches were prepared making sure that we had something from each food group *daily*. At home, my parents also cooked full course meals that included each food group. As we get older and grow up, many of us tend to stray away from the importance of the four food groups and their nutritional concept. So many people began to abandon exercising and then later find themselves gaining weight and becoming more susceptible to health problems. There is a higher diagnosis rate of diseases and ailments than ever. Eating microwave foods and microwave dinners that are processed and acidic has become the norm for many people that are in a rush. Due to the infamous microwave, many healthy full course meals we grew up with have taken a backseat in a lot of the kitchens and homes across our country.

On page two of this publication in the disclaimer, I asked the reader to think about consuming their foods without always using a microwave. I am not telling anyone to never use microwaves, I am just asking that you pull away from it for a minute to see if your health improves. Your meal may have been nutritious at first but would heating your food in the microwave strip away it's original nutrients? Could microwaving cause your dinner to change into dead food due to the the molecular structure in your food changing? The health benefits of vitamin B12 and a few other B vitamins could be lowered if heated in a microwave. One study showed there was a 30% - 40% loss of the much needed vitamin B12 when the foods received microwave exposure. Another study found that spinach retained nearly all of it's *folate* in the microwave but lost about 77% of it on the stove. Cooking food in a lot of water can destroy many water soluble vitamins. I often steam or eat my produce in their most natural state. If you experience irregular heart beat or any chest pain, you definitely may need to be careful if you use a microwave on a consistent basis. On pg 139, you will see where I discussed the potential harm microwaving foods while they are wrapped in plastic could cause. I use the oven more than I use the microwave. Always do what's best for you.

Just a slight reminder, the #1 salad I mentioned in the Multiple Sclerosis section on page 37 has each one of the four food groups in it. The sub sandwich I mentioned on page 39 will also provide all four food groups. The #1 - #8 options blessed me with great health improvements and guaranteed me that victory was attainable. Eating foods individually is fine but eating them together will certainly provide added positive results. For best results, try eating foods from each food group each day and consume your produce raw and fresh (Also see end of pg 111).

"Fresh daily" salads from a reputable location where the salad can breathe appear to improve my health more than bagged salads found in grocery stores. Salads constantly have light and oxygen in most restaurants. Oxygen repairs cells, contracts our muscles, calms our nerves and feeds our brain. I often add 35g of grilled chicken to my salads.

2016 UPDATE

I know that I mention MS a lot but hey, that's my diagnosis. I have been trying to research B13 since the latter 90s after I read it could possibly help aid MS sufferers. The limited information that I found back then stated B13 could be found in the liquid portion of curdled milk (*whey*) and root vegetables such as garlic, potatoes, onions, beets and carrots. I prefer the first ingredient in my cheese to be whey. Whey has been very instrumental to my recovery. Today there is still not a lot of information on B13. It may not be recognized as a vitamin but it is very important. B13 can help assist in the absorption of calcium, magnesium and essential nutrients. It can metabolize *folate* and vitamin B12. B13 is created by the body by intestinal flora. Feed your intestinal probiotics with prebiotics to increase your healthy intestinal flora. Probiotics can change your life.

Probiotics increase the flora in your body. Easily found in fermented food: ACV, kefir, kimchi, miso, sauerkraut, kombucha/green tea, soy sauce, yogurt

Prebiotics are the food for intestinal flora growth. Garlic, onions, bread, whole grains, apples, honey, beans, bananas, cocoa, mushrooms, okra, seaweed

Avoid the things that will destroy your healthy intestinal flora. *Stress, excess sugar, alcohol, many medications, artificial food coloring, chlorinated drinking water, synthetic laxatives and poor diet (fast food, processed foods)* are enemies that could harm or destroy your intestinal flora.

I am a strong believer in consuming my produce fresh and in their most natural state. However, I can not leave off the fermented vegetables. They can provide numerous health benefits as well. The beneficial bacteria in fermented foods are very potent detoxifiers. They are capable of drawing out a wide range of toxins and heavy metals such as mercury, lead, aluminum and arsenates. You do not need to consume large amounts to reap the benefits either. *One quarter to one ½ of a cup of fermented foods each day can strengthen your intestinal gut.* Having the appropriate balance of gut bacteria and digestive enzymes will help the body better absorb the nutrients found in the foods consumed. I try to keep my intestinal flora healthy and strong because I want all vitamins and minerals absorbed from my diet. (Darker miso has been fermented the longest.)

Top fermented choices: sauerkraut, kefir, kimchi, kombucha tea, miso soup and real yogurt. Kefir is *superior to yogurt.* I prefer my sauerkraut salt-free, unpasteurized and unheated. I will never heat the sauerkraut because heat will destroy the enzymes and valuable probiotics. Fermented vegetables can help balance your stomach acid by raising stomach acid if it is to low, then lowering it if the acid is to high. They encourage proper HCL production. On page 41, I explained how important the production of HCL is for improved health. Make sure when you buy your fermented vegetables you are buying quality and not something pasteurized or packed in vinegar and salt. The production of HCL is vital to proper digestion and achieving optimal health.

Dysfunction of our brain is normally connected to what is happening in our intestines. Your digestive system serves as your second brain. Various health symptoms in our body originate from our digestive system. Fermented foods help us with brain health, depression and anxiety. The greater the variety of fermented and cultured foods you have in your diet the better. Eating fermented foods produce more of the *neurotransmitter* serotonin. Serotonin is known to have a positive influence on a person's mood. A variety of fermented foods provide many different microorganisms for our stomach. **Most cheeses** are fermented **but** cheddar, cottage, feta, Gouda, hoop, Parmesan and provolone **also** have vital probiotics. (Red Miso: aged longer than white or yellow miso)

In my first book *My MS Success,* I was constantly studying and trying to achieve the Diet #1 status. That's the health status I achieved in the ladder 90s where I felt great and the closest to 100% after my MS diagnosis. On page 31 in this book, I share my recent main options that assisted me in great health on my job for more than 13 yrs. In 2016 I was able to get my best understanding on what was possibly assisting my health in the latter 90s. On page 146 you will see a part that says Brain Function in the vitamin K section. It tells you *myelin sheath* needs sphingolipids (**s-fing-go-lipids**) to properly form. Sphingolipids help inhibit cholesterol absorption and synthesis in the intestine and they help protect against colon cancer. Sphingolipids are involved in intracellular signaling from the cell exterior to the cell interior. *Cell communication* is very important.

In the Western diet, sphingolipids are calculated to be about 0.01 - 0.02% of the diet. **That is a very small amount.** The most common dietary sources where most people get their sphingolipids are from dairy products. They are found in small amounts so I list food sources that provide the most per mg/kg based on my understanding and studies. Although a lot of studies and research has been done, I found very limited data on sphingolipids at the time I was able to study them in 2016. There's more than 300 complex sphingolipids. (A fat-soluble molecule derived from amino acid with an unsaturated hydrocarbon chain.)

Cereal: durum wheat flour 198, wheat flour 158, rye flour 151, rye grains 123, oat flakes 84

Dairy: butter 1170, cream 907 (cream is normally 1st or 2nd ingredient in **natural** ice cream), cheese 567 (I want **whey** as my 1st cheese ingredient), butter-milk 292

Eggs: 2250 cook your eggs, raw is harder to digest
I read a report:1 in every 30,000 eggs **may** have salmonella

Fish: salmon 301, herring 184, cod 118

Meat:chicken 589, lamb 498, turkey 497, beef 448

Vegetables: soy beans 2410 (**red miso** offers the **most vital** fermented soy beans), sweet potato 669, soy flour 601, fava beans 502, kidney beans 412, peas 369

NOTE: Natural ice cream normally has 5-7 ingredients. Natural butter normally has 2-3 ingredients. Natural ice cream and butter do not have a lot of extra ingredients.

On page 173, I introduced *"The Clevon Diet"*. I explained the D in CED stands for Diet. We need to watch what we eat *(avoid inflammatory food pg 166)*. Limit or eliminate some of the foods below. If you do this, your health status will "Thank you!" The foods I limited or stayed away from to achieve success are below.(Drink coffee/tea **1 hr** after eating.) 1. Coffee **(**Over consumption can result in depleted calcium, magnesium and decrease iron absorption. Magnesium works with calcium and vitamin D to aid in energy production and facilitate the muscle contraction/relaxation response. Look over the **MS Health Chart** on pg 124 in *My Ms Success*. Excess sugar in coffee can easily disrupt that Chart's plan. **Never drink coffee or tea on an empty stomach.)**

2. Cake

3. Candy

4. Chips

5. Cookies

6. Doughnuts

7. Fast Food

8. French Fries

9. Fried Foods

10. Ice Cream (I like vanilla. Vanilla bean can fight *inflammation*, cancer, cholesterol, anxiety & acne.)

11. Soda

12. Sweet Juices

13. White Bread

RECAP AND FINALE

I drink Isopure isolated *whey* protein on an **empty stomach**, 1-2 hours before I eat, after I exercise for muscle repair or *gradually* during the day. Strive to *perform jumping exercises such as jumping jacks, jump roping or jump lunges daily. This strengthens our cardio.* Lactic acid is produced when strenuous exercise depletes our oxygen. If you take Isopure, I suggest exercising with it for best results. I usually eat something with *a little fat* later on to absorb the fat-soluble vitamins Isopure has. Your HCL can be strengthened by eating beans. High amounts of B1, B2, B6, E, K, C, iron, zinc, calcium, phosphorous, protein, potassium, magnesium, manganese, folate and fiber are found in **beans**. See page 96, 178

Kellogg's Total, brewer's or nutritional yeast and raw wheat germ have a lot of B1, *folate*, etc. B1 repairs our *myelin* and *immune system.* Pg 156,173

Phosphorous helps transference of *nerve impulses.* **Source:** *beef, fish, poultry, milk, egg, cheese,beans*

I credit a lot of my Diet #1 status in the late 90s to the foods on page 56. I ate **most** of them daily. I subconsciously ate *selenium, lycopene,* in addition to *carnitine, tyrosine, zinc* and *salt. Carnitine* and *tyrosine* (**sources:** beef, chicken, fish) aid in *faster muscle reflexes.* I continue to consume *whey* (B13), *folate, sphingolipids,* salad, fish, iron and I feed my intestinal flora (pg 206). I eat enzyme/alkaline/anti-inflammatory food daily. Magnesium, turmeric and fulvic are consumed often. (***Mushrooms are easier absorbed and healthier when grilled or microwaved.***)

L-Tyrosine is synthetic. Tyrosine is an amino acid produced in our bodies naturally by the amino acid phenylalanine. Tyrosine improves focus, alertness, attention, aids in faster reflexes and produces brain chemicals that allow nerve cells to communicate. Tyrosine was first discovered in cheese. In Greek, *Tyros* means *cheese*. (*Tyrosine is copious in Swiss & Romano cheese, Calcium lactate in cheddar & Colby.*)

Tyrosine: steak (skirt), pork chop, salmon, chicken breast, turkey, soy/tofu, milk, cheese, beans, tuna See page 40, 64, 76 (#6 and #8), 102 and page 135

Carnitine: whey protein, red meat, pork, milk, cod

Eat with carbs to absorb into your muscle cells. pg 174

I often mix milk and 3 tbsp of nutritional yeast. pg 156

Phenylalanine: steak, chicken breast, pork chops, tofu, tuna, pinto beans, milk, sweet potatoes, eggs

B6, **Copper** or **Folate** assist in tyrosine absorption.

Dopamine (pg 2) needs tyrosine. Avoid extra sugar.

If you want quality films, videos, graphic designs, CDs, etc contact Jude Boi Films today.
JudeBoiFilms.Com or call 256 947 2189

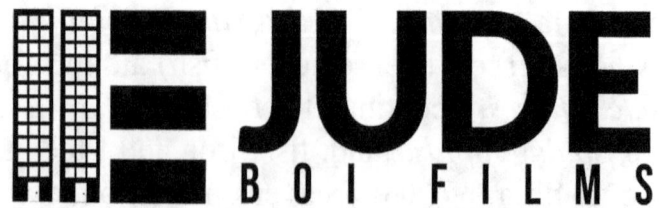

--ANYTHING IS POSSIBLE TO THOSE WHO BELIEVE--

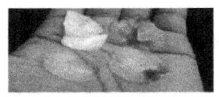

NOVELc Supplement   (4 Vons above.)

My personal/trusted Novelc supplement is found on page 108 and 180. I was definitely in the first or second grade when I learned how to make it. This supplement was taken to protect us all from serious viruses. It didn't require taking much. After mother handed me one, I secretly made and took another because I liked the taste of it. It is now decades later and I "still" have "never" been infected with a serious virus. I can't recall my siblings getting very sick either. I have been around many sick/infected people, some questioned why I never got infected. Even though I never took a flu shot, I never caught the flu either. Decades later, my mom noticed that I had Vons made. She asked if she could have one. I had forgotten that she takes her blood pressure and cholesterol medicine. I thank God she had zero bad side-effects. I don't know anyone that has taken it and had negative side-effects. Ingredients required to make it sounds strange but I am doing fine and I am ready to take it again if asked or feel I need to. I love how this is not government made or political and I can make them myself. After all these years, it appears viruses can't reside in my body for long. I mentioned this supplement back in 2004 but later removed it from that publication because for some reason, I felt it was not time. Remember, I 1st made and took this supplement when I was a child. That has been almost 4 decades ago. Every Von will not look identical. This book is about good health, so I shared it here. Novelc gave me positive, enduring and expeditious results. Lisa had no more ER visits and her ejection fraction went from 10% - 50%. I'm not sure what all Novelc does but it does a lot. I'm still stunned. She takes 15-20 medicines a day and had zero side-effects. I tried sharing the order sheet Lisa gave me consent to reveal below, to verify her congestive heart failure. (FDA suggested I call my product a supplement and give it a name. I named it Novelc. It's novel! Von, pg 1. I filed for a patent.)

9/5/2022 3:52 PM   https://visiontm.netsmartcloud.com/Web1/Reports/RptPhysOrders_20425_20229251455226_1.htm

September 2022 Physician Order Sheet

Print Date: 9/25/2022 2:52:26 PM

Order / Medication(s)	Frequency
Calcium Carbonate 400 mg calcium (1,000 mg) chewable tablet (2) TABLET CHEWABLE Oral	Two Times Daily Starting 09/15/2022
Lansoprazole ... TYPE 2 DIABETES MELLITUS WITH DIABETIC CHRONIC KIDNEY DISEASE	Every One Day Starting 09/15/2022
Ofloxacin 0.3 % eye drops (4-5 gtts) DROPS Left Ear; Instructions: Ofloxacin 0.3% solution 4-5 gtts to affected ear(s) bid x 7 days. OTITIS EXTERNA, LEFT EAR	Two Times Daily for Seven Days Starting 09/22/2022
Ramelteon 7.5mg CAPSULE Oral; Instructions: Ramelteon 7.5mg QHS. Therapeutic Range: INSOMNIA, UNSPECIFIED	Hour Of Sleep Starting 09/23/2022

9/5/2022 2:43 PM   https://visiontm.netsmartcloud.com/Web1/Reports/RptPhysOrders_20425_20229251455226_1.htm

September 2022 Physician Order Sheet

Print Date: 9/25/2022 2:43 PM

Order / Medication(s)	Frequency
Amoxicillin 500 mg capsule (2) CAPSULE Oral by mouth every day x3weeks. Instructions: . Therapeutic Range:	Every One Day Starting 08/26/2022
Dicyclomine 10 mg capsule (1 cap) CAPSULE Oral by mouth twice daily as needed for abdominal pain. Instructions: . Therapeutic Range: IRRITABLE BOWEL SYNDROME WITH CONSTIPATION	As Needed Two Times Daily Starting 08/25/2022
Ondansetron 8 mg disintegrating tablet (1 tablet) TABLET,DISINTEGRATING Oral by mouth every 12 hrs PRN for nausea/ vomiting. Instructions: . Therapeutic Range:	As Needed Every Twelve Hours Starting 08/25/2022
Spironolactone 25 mg tablet (0.5 tab) TABLET Oral Instructions: 0.5 - 12.5 mg per dose. Therapeutic Range: CHRONIC COMBINED SYSTOLIC (CONGESTIVE) AND DIASTOLIC (CONGESTIVE) HEART FAILURE	Every One Day Starting 08/25/2022
Temazepam 15 mg capsule (1) CAPSULE Oral 15mg capsule qhs for insomnia. Instructions: . Therapeutic Range: INSOMNIA, UNSPECIFIED	Hour Of Sleep Starting 09/07/2022

Patient Name	PatID	Location	Patient Sex	Patient Date of Birth	Admission ID	Admission Date	Page Number
Gardner, Lisa	191101	A/104/100H/Sta 1/Millennium/Region 6/THM	Female	12/24/1966	Mil. 70796	6/30/2021	3 continued

My dream and desire is for a reputable company to study and mass produce my Novelc supplement. As I prepare to close, I want to say thank you to those who support their loved ones that are/may be suffering during a time they need you most. Some feel deserted and some are frustrated. We love you! Special thank you to Mr. Jamaal Jude for my cover design, Mr. Bolsinger for his informative help and thank you the reader for taking the time to read this publication. I pray the reader will be blessed with knowledge & prosper with optimal health. I thank God for his many blessings. May God bless you!!! **"Life is more enjoyable when you are healthy!"**

Job 11:18

*And thou shalt be secure, because there is hope; yea, thou shalt dig **about thee, and** thou shalt take thy rest in safety.*

King James Version

Job 11:18

Having hope will give you courage. You will be protected and will rest in safety.

New Living Translation

Jeremiah 33:3

Call unto me, and I will answer thee, and shew thee great and mighty things, which thou knowest not.

II Corinthians 12:10

Therefore I take pleasure in infirmities, in reproaches, in necessities, in persecutions, in distresses for Christ's sake: for when I am weak, then am I strong.

(1 tsp/turmeric, dash of pepper plus 8**oz** water heals & see page **2**. Talk to a doctor before changing your diet.)